Limerick City and County Library

3 0027 00895237 3

D1765524

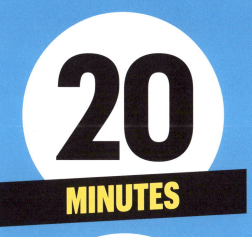

20
MINUTES

4
WEEKS

1
DYNAMITE BODY!

Tone & Trim
in No Time

JANET LEE

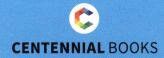

CENTENNIAL BOOKS

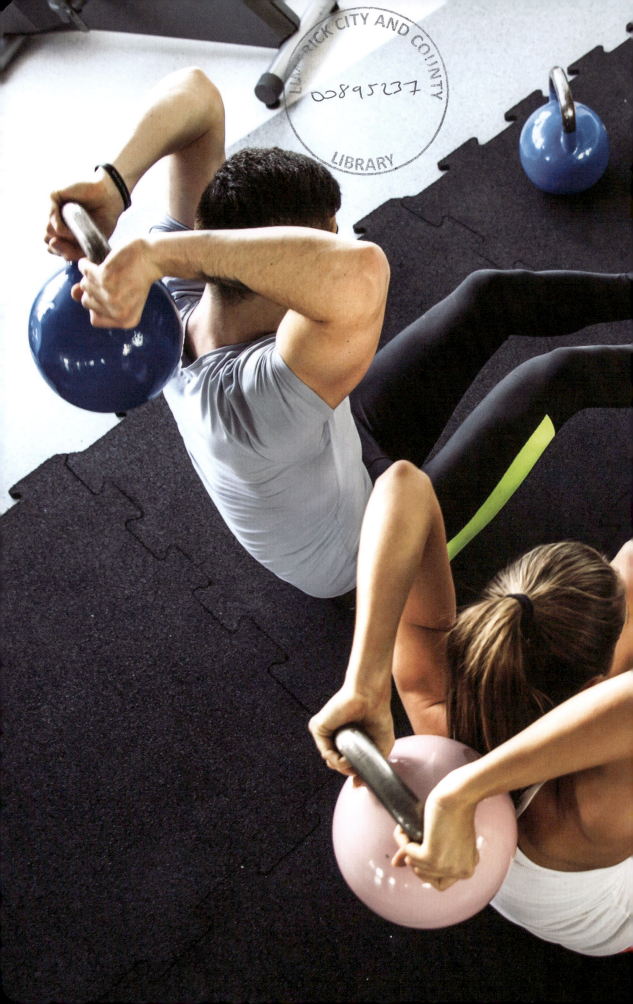
LIMERICK CITY AND COUNTY
00895237
LIBRARY

20
MINUTES

4
WEEKS

1
DYNAMITE BODY!

Tone & Trim in No Time

CONTENTS

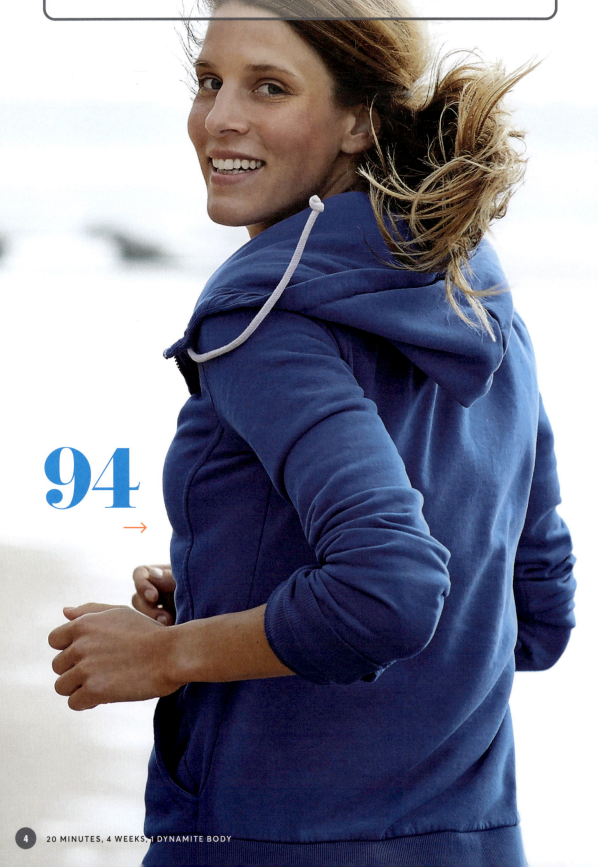

94
→

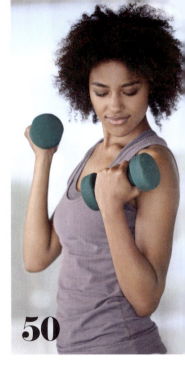

50

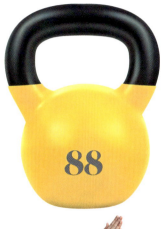

88

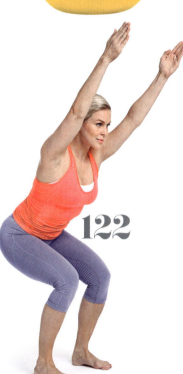

122

The 20-Minute Strategy

Yes, you do have time to get strong and healthy in just minutes a day!

Nutrition and exercise: They're the ultimate healthy duo. They have a huge impact on how you feel, how well your body and brain work, and even how long you live—not to mention how you look. If you can dial them in, you may be able to avoid various conditions, including type 2 diabetes, high cholesterol, hypertension and depression. You're nodding. You get it. You're working on the diet—you have to eat, after all—but sometimes exercise is just so hard to squeeze in. Changing, driving to the gym, showering, not to mention figuring out what to do. It's time-consuming and, well, a little boring.

But exercise doesn't have to be that complicated (or mind-numbing). For health benefits, all you need to accumulate is 30 minutes of moderate-intensity cardio five days a week—or 21 minutes daily. Just 21 minutes! (If you take up the intensity, you can get by with less.) Of course, you need some weight training too, because that's the secret sauce for maintaining or losing weight, looking and feeling lean and firm, and fitting into the clothes you love, especially as you age. Before your mind starts spiraling about how you'll fit *that* in too, don't worry. Combining cardio and strength is the *extra* secret sauce. It saves time, adds intensity and works your whole body. And finally, there's the "what to do?" part. Nobody wants to bang out the same workout day after day; variety is good for your muscles and noggin. That's why you need this book.

Here's What to Expect in the Pages Ahead:

▶ **FAST AND EFFICIENT WORKOUTS** The 20-minute routines here—whether cardio, HIIT, strength or a combo—are laid out for you, move by move and minute by minute. Best of all, you can do them in your own home, at the park, at the gym or wherever you want.

▶ **TOTAL-BODY TONE-UPS** There are strength exercises to work every area of your body, including key muscle groups like your arms, abs, legs and butt.

▶ **EQUIPMENT-FREE EXERCISES** You'll find moves that involve your body weight only, as well as routines that use basic tools, such as dumbbells, bands, balls or kettlebells. You don't need a ton of gear to get the job done!

▶ **BOREDOM-BUSTING CARDIO** It runs the gamut from moderate to way-intense and involves hills, circuits, intervals and even yoga. You won't be doing the same thing for 20 minutes, guaranteed! You'll burn serious calories and fat to get leaner faster.

▶ **RESTORATIVE STRETCHES** Make nice with your muscles on your off days (or even post-workout) with some easy stretching.

▶ **MIX-AND-MATCH PROGRAMMING** Flexibility is built in. If you have more time you can combine workouts, and if you want to change the level, it's easy to add or remove rest time to suit your energy. No excuses!

Ready to see how much you can accomplish in just 20 minutes? Let's move! —*Janet Lee*

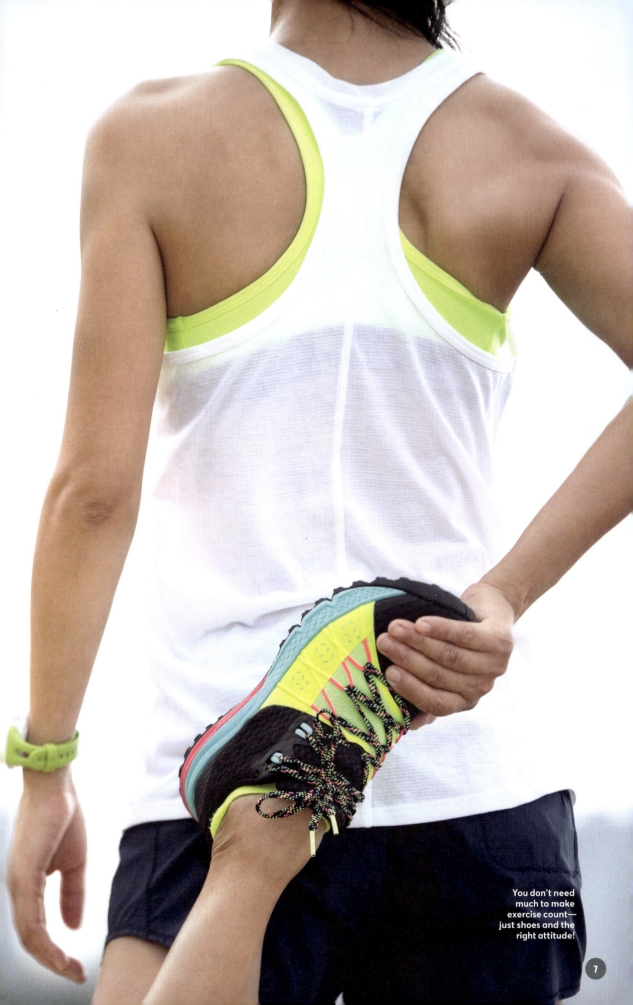

You don't need
much to make
exercise count—
just shoes and the
right attitude!

28 Days to Dynamite!

Use this structured program if you want a set routine to keep you on track.

Exercise doesn't have to be complicated. The chart and calendar here show you exactly how you can put together the cardio, strength and interval routines in this book without spending a ton of time getting it done. If a workout calls for a machine or equipment you don't have, use what you do have, or pick another routine in the same category that works for you. You'll find these exercises beginning on page 50.

C = CARDIO
S = STRENGTH
I = INTENSE CARDIO
M = CARDIO/STRENGTH COMBO
R = RECOVERY

WEEK 1

▶ **DAY 1** Outdoor Circuit
▶ **DAY 2** HIIT Workout (pick any plan)
▶ **DAY 3** Strong From Head to Toe
▶ **DAY 4** Hill Workout (pick any plan)
▶ **DAY 5** Rest Day or Yoga Flow
▶ **DAY 6** Boot Camp Blast
▶ **DAY 7** The STEM Program

C I S I R I S M

WEEK 2

▶ **DAY 8** Machine Circuit
▶ **DAY 9** Get With the Band
▶ **DAY 10** Rest Day or Stretch Goals
▶ **DAY 11** Strength Circuit
▶ **DAY 12** Flat Abs Fast (pick any plan)
▶ **DAY 13** HIIT Workout (pick any plan)
▶ **DAY 14** Saved By the Bell

C S R M S I S

WEEK 3

▶ **DAY 15** Rest Day or Yoga Flow
▶ **DAY 16** Hill Workout (pick any plan)
▶ **DAY 17** Welcome to the Gun Show
▶ **DAY 18** HIIT Combo Circuit
▶ **DAY 19** Plump Your Peach
▶ **DAY 20** Rest Day or Yoga Flow
▶ **DAY 21** Outdoor Circuit

R I S I S R C

WEEK 4

▶ **DAY 22** Have a Ball!
▶ **DAY 23** HIIT Workout (pick any plan)
▶ **DAY 24** Get With the Band
▶ **DAY 25** Rest Day or Stretch Goals
▶ **DAY 26** Strong to the Core
▶ **DAY 27** Boot Camp Blast
▶ **DAY 28** Pair Up for Super Results

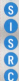

S I S R S I M S

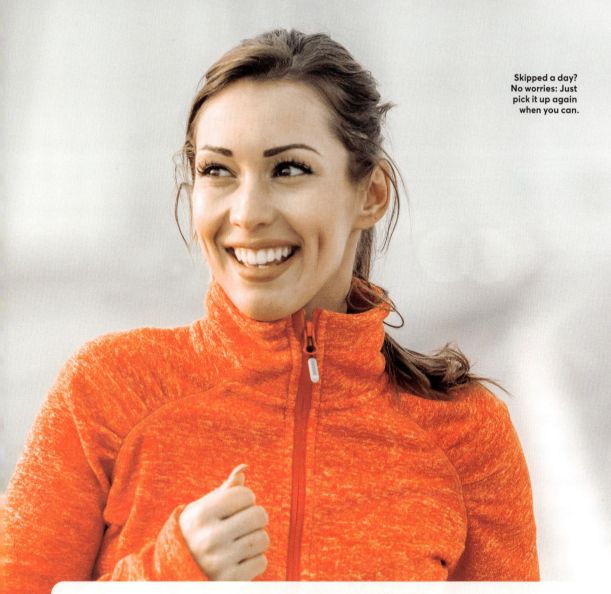

Skipped a day? No worries: Just pick it up again when you can.

4 WEEKS TO FAB

SUNDAY	MONDAY	TUESDAY	WEDNESDAY	THURSDAY	FRIDAY	SATURDAY
Outdoor Circuit **C**	HIIT Workout (pick any plan) **I**	Strong From Head to Toe **S**	Hill Workout (pick any plan) **I**	Rest Day or Yoga Flow **R**	Boot Camp Blast **I M**	The STEM Program **S**
Machine Circuit **C**	Get With the Band **S**	Rest Day or Stretch Goals **R**	Strength Circuit **M**	Flat Abs Fast (pick any plan) **S**	HIIT Workout (pick any plan) **I**	Saved By the Bell **S**
Rest Day or Yoga Flow **R**	Hill Workout (pick any plan) **I**	Welcome to the Gun Show **S**	HIIT Combo Circuit **I**	Plump Your Peach **S**	Rest Day or Yoga Flow **R**	Outdoor Circuit **C**
Have a Ball! **S**	HIIT Workout (pick any plan) **I**	Get With the Band **S**	Rest Day or Stretch Goals **R**	Strong to the Core **S**	Boot Camp Blast **I M**	Pair Up for Super Results **S**

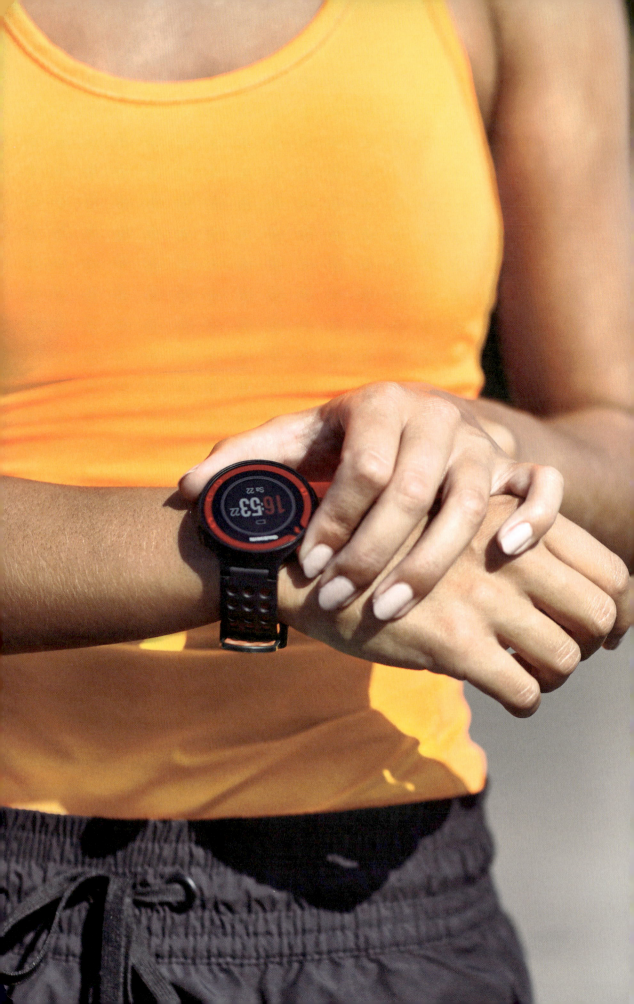

THE BASICS

↓

Exercise Is Medicine

BEING PHYSICALLY ACTIVE IS ONE OF THE BEST THINGS YOU CAN DO FOR YOUR BRAIN AND BODY. A WELL-ROUNDED ROUTINE WITH CARDIO, WEIGHTS AND STRETCHING WILL HELP KEEP YOU FEELING YOUNGER LONGER AND REDUCE THE RISK OF ILLNESS. OUR PROGRAM COVERS ALL THE BASES.

Exercise: The Ultimate Rx for Health

Physical activity is the proverbial fountain of youth.

The old saying "Let food be thy medicine…"—from Hippocrates circa 400 B.C.—needs a modern update: Let food *and* regular exercise be thy medicine. Tons of research has shown how moving more, and doing so on a consistent basis, helps reduce the risk of a variety of diseases and can even help treat certain health conditions. "Getting 150 minutes a week [of aerobic exercise] is clearly enough to prevent a number of diseases and conditions, including coronary heart disease, high blood pressure, stroke, type 2 diabetes, metabolic syndrome, colon cancer, breast cancer and depression, as well as all-cause mortality and falls and declines in cognitive function," says Judith Regensteiner, PhD, professor of medicine and director of the center for women's health research at the University of Colorado School of Medicine. "There's probably a point below that amount that is effective, too. Anything is better than nothing." (And more is better than anything.) There's not a single pill out there—prescription or over-the-counter—that does that. Imagine how much it would cost if there were? You can get all this for free!

Here's the best part: You don't have to carve an hour out of your schedule and slog away on the treadmill or weight machines. Who has time for that? You can get a perfectly good workout and knock off both cardio and strength work in just 20 minutes. On the following pages we'll explain the basics about exercise, why it's so important, and how to use this issue to guide you, whether you're a newbie or trying to change it up. Turn the page to get started!

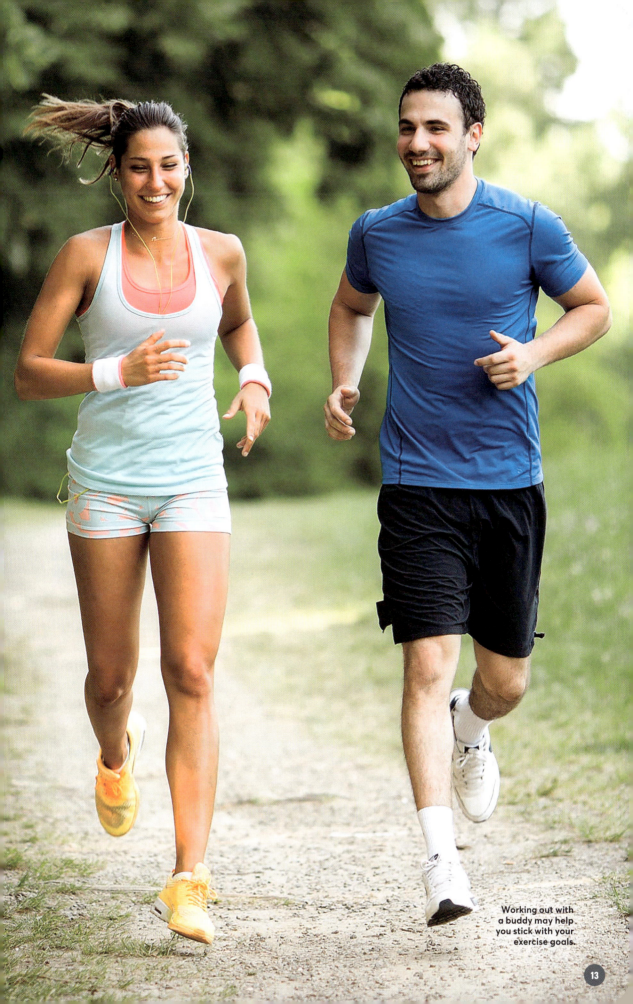

Working out with a buddy may help you stick with your exercise goals.

What Does It Take?

Every so often a group of exercise researchers from the American College of Sports Medicine (ACSM) gets together to look at reams of data about how exercise impacts health. The resulting Position Stand lays out exactly how much exercise you need to see health benefits (not necessarily for weight loss or big fitness improvements). They've determined that the following have well-documented benefits for adults of all ages:

▶ **150 MINUTES** of moderate-intensity cardio exercise a week—or about half that amount if it's vigorous

▶ **2 OR 3** strength-training workouts a week that target your entire body (arms, shoulders, chest, back, abs, butt and legs)

▶ **2 OR 3** flexibility sessions a week that target your entire body

▶ **2 OR 3** neuromotor exercise training sessions a week (that includes things like balance, agility and gait training, and yoga)

Know Your "Meds"

Just like taking pills, you should know what you're getting, how it's affecting your body and how to take it.

CARDIO This is shorthand for aerobic (and sometimes beyond) exercise. It means anything from walking to high-intensity interval training (HIIT). This kind of exercise

21–32%

Ideal body fat percentage for an adult woman

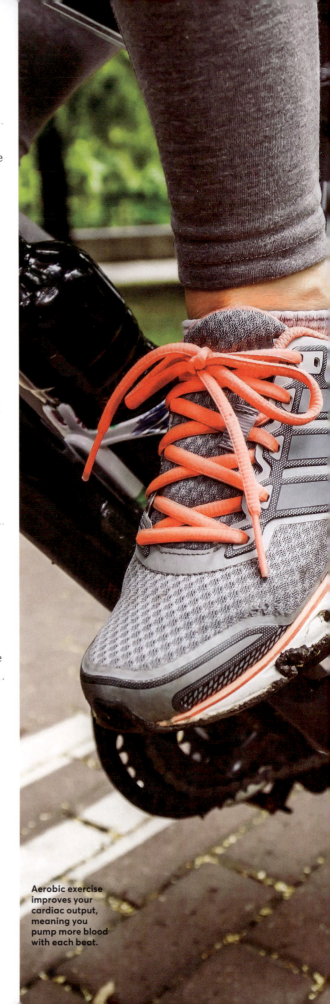

Aerobic exercise improves your cardiac output, meaning you pump more blood with each beat.

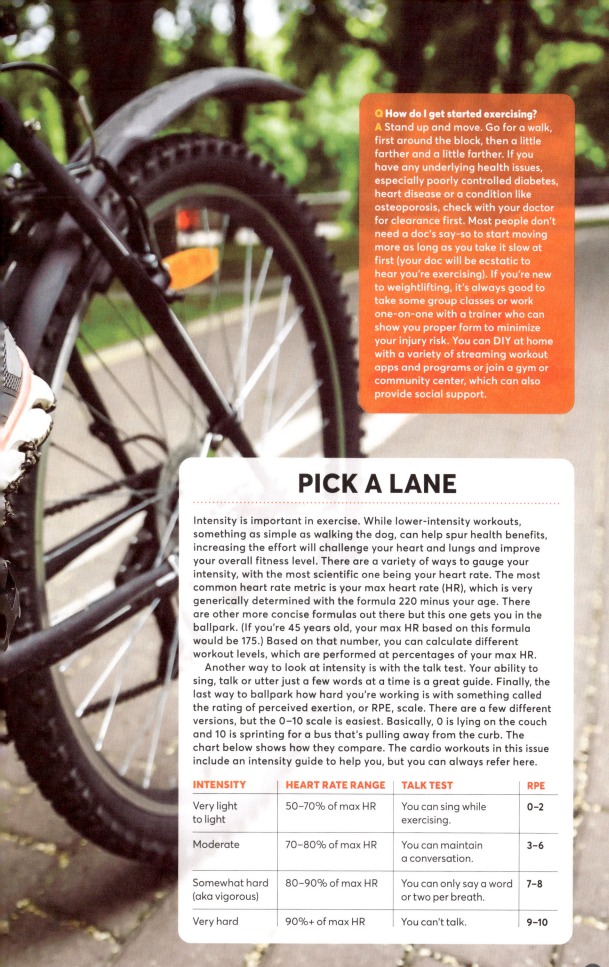

Q How do I get started exercising?
A Stand up and move. Go for a walk, first around the block, then a little farther and a little farther. If you have any underlying health issues, especially poorly controlled diabetes, heart disease or a condition like osteoporosis, check with your doctor for clearance first. Most people don't need a doc's say-so to start moving more as long as you take it slow at first (your doc will be ecstatic to hear you're exercising). If you're new to weightlifting, it's always good to take some group classes or work one-on-one with a trainer who can show you proper form to minimize your injury risk. You can DIY at home with a variety of streaming workout apps and programs or join a gym or community center, which can also provide social support.

PICK A LANE

Intensity is important in exercise. While lower-intensity workouts, something as simple as walking the dog, can help spur health benefits, increasing the effort will challenge your heart and lungs and improve your overall fitness level. There are a variety of ways to gauge your intensity, with the most scientific one being your heart rate. The most common heart rate metric is your max heart rate (HR), which is very generically determined with the formula 220 minus your age. There are other more concise formulas out there but this one gets you in the ballpark. (If you're 45 years old, your max HR based on this formula would be 175.) Based on that number, you can calculate different workout levels, which are performed at percentages of your max HR.

Another way to look at intensity is with the talk test. Your ability to sing, talk or utter just a few words at a time is a great guide. Finally, the last way to ballpark how hard you're working is with something called the rating of perceived exertion, or RPE, scale. There are a few different versions, but the 0–10 scale is easiest. Basically, 0 is lying on the couch and 10 is sprinting for a bus that's pulling away from the curb. The chart below shows how they compare. The cardio workouts in this issue include an intensity guide to help you, but you can always refer here.

INTENSITY	HEART RATE RANGE	TALK TEST	RPE
Very light to light	50–70% of max HR	You can sing while exercising.	0–2
Moderate	70–80% of max HR	You can maintain a conversation.	3–6
Somewhat hard (aka vigorous)	80–90% of max HR	You can only say a word or two per breath.	7–8
Very hard	90%+ of max HR	You can't talk.	9–10

challenges your heart and lungs, training them to get stronger and more efficient. That delivers many of the health benefits listed earlier but also has impacts on mood and brain function and may impact how your cells age.

The ACSM recommends accumulating 30 minutes or more of moderate exercise five days a week, or 20 minutes or more of vigorous exercise three days a week. That's how powerful higher-intensity workouts are. Can't carve out 20 minutes or more? You can accumulate this time in 10-minute bursts (or even less than that) if necessary; the goal is to just move as often as you can. (See Chapter 3 for a variety of cardio workouts, including hills, intervals, circuits and more.)

STRENGTH TRAINING Also known as resistance or weight training, it involves using your body weight or some other type of resistance to challenge your muscles and make them stronger. Even though the focus is your muscles, strength training has benefits for your heart and reduces your overall risk of dying early. It's also good for improving blood pressure and blood sugar levels and can help strengthen bones. (See Chapter 2 for a variety of resistance exercises that target every major muscle group.)

Resistance might include dumbbells, exercise tubing, barbells, weight machines, kettlebells and more. Generally, you want to aim for three to four sets of eight to 12 repetitions using a weight that feels challenging to lift with good form by that last repetition. If you go slightly lighter with the weight, aim for 10 to 15 reps. Research has shown you can get by just fine with one or two sets, but a new study published in the journal *Sports Medicine* found that, in women, the more often they lifted (especially if it was three or more days a week), the more strength they gained. The individual variables (weight, reps) weren't as important.

FLEXIBILITY TRAINING Stretching after a workout is a good way to cool down and boost range of motion, which can decline with age. Target your entire body and hold each stretch for 10 to 30 seconds. There are many different approaches to flexibility work; we're keeping it pretty straightforward in this issue. (See Chapter 4 for some easy stretching routines.)

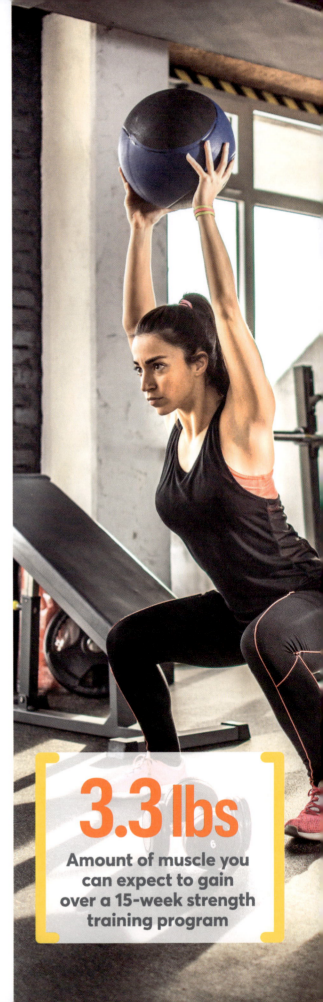

3.3 lbs [6]

Amount of muscle you can expect to gain over a 15-week strength training program

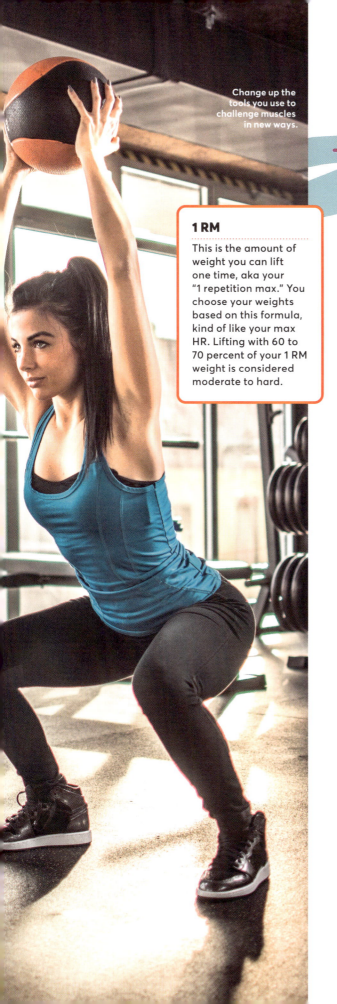

Change up the tools you use to challenge muscles in new ways.

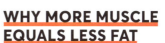

1 RM

This is the amount of weight you can lift one time, aka your "1 repetition max." You choose your weights based on this formula, kind of like your max HR. Lifting with 60 to 70 percent of your 1 RM weight is considered moderate to hard.

WHY MORE MUSCLE EQUALS LESS FAT

▶ Many people get this equation wrong. "Women get focused on burning calories when they're trying to lose weight. They're avoiding the weights," says trainer David Freeman, the national brand manager for the Alpha small group training class at Life Time. "As a result, they're losing muscle, which increases their body fat percentage." When you cut calories significantly (or increase the amount you're burning), your body can easily decide to tap into muscle stores for the energy it needs. But if you lose muscle, you're sabotaging your ability to keep that weight off. While both muscle and fat cells burn a relatively small number of calories just hanging around on your body, muscle burns way more than fat. If you lose muscle, your metabolism, which will already slow down as you get lighter, will be even slower. Wrong move! Adding muscle by strength training will help keep that metabolism revved, ensuring that the weight that comes off is from fat. Plus, a pound of muscle is more compact than a pound of fat. It takes up less space, so your physique changes even if the scale does not.

The Big 2-0

If you take the ACSM's 150-minute weekly exercise recommendation and divide it by 7, it comes out to approximately 21.5 minutes a day. That seems pretty doable, right? The trick to maximizing that time is to be focused and keep moving. The 20-minute workouts in this book were created with just that intention in mind: Get in, get out. They're so speedy you could even do two or three a day if you're motivated. Here's what you'll find in this book:

CHAPTER 1 includes all the foundational exercise info you need to get started, from the importance of adding in rest and active recovery days to surprising exercise myths and the best ways to fuel up for your workouts.

CHAPTER 2 is all about strength training. The workouts are designed to be doable at home with only a few pieces of equipment. You can find everything you need at a local retail store like Target or Walmart, or you can order online. The exercises in this section target your entire body in multiple ways. They're designed to be done with no more than a minute of rest between moves. Some plans also offer ways to cut out or minimize the amount of rest you'll take and "cardio-fy" it with aerobic or high-energy bursts. You're turning a strength workout into a cardio *and* strength session. (Yes, you can double-dip.) Take it at your speed. If you need to rest, then rest. If you want to challenge yourself, go for it.

CHAPTER 3 contains a dozen cardio workouts, from circuits to hills to high-intensity intervals. Some are more moderate intensity (a conversational level), but most will be at the "somewhat hard" level (hard to speak more than a few words). For the most diversity, you'll need a workout machine like a treadmill or stationary bike, but you could do many of them outdoors on a walk or jog or with a bicycle.

CHAPTER 4 features some yoga and basic stretching routines to help you limber up in different ways. It's easiest to stretch after your regular workout, but you don't have to.

SCHEDULE YOURSELF

Here's how all this might look when broken down on a weekly calendar. You can accumulate both moderate and vigorous exercise to reach your weekly goal; it's not a matter of either/or. (Every minute of vigorous exercise counts as two moderate minutes, more or less.) Find our full 4-week plan on page 8.

	MONDAY	TUESDAY	WEDNESDAY	THURSDAY	FRIDAY	SATURDAY	SUNDAY
EXERCISE	Cardio	Strength (upper or lower body or total body). Do it fast and call it cardio, too.	Cardio (make one day a week a longer— say, 45 minutes— moderate-paced session)	Strength (total body)	Cardio (HIIT or hills)	Strength (upper or lower body or total body). Do it fast and call it cardio, too.	Stretch or Yoga Flow
DURATION	20 mins.	20 mins.	45 mins.	20 mins.	20 mins.	20 mins.	20 mins.
INTENSITY	Moderate	Vigorous	Moderate	Moderate	Vigorous	Vigorous	Easy

Cardio (we're counting strength if it's fast): 125 minutes over 5 sessions. How it breaks down:
Moderate 65 minutes
Vigorous 60 minutes (This is the equivalent of 120 moderate-intensity minutes. Add these to your 65 minutes above and you're over your 150-minute moderate-intensity goal!)
Strength 3 sessions
Stretch 1 long stretch plus 5 to 10 minutes after every session

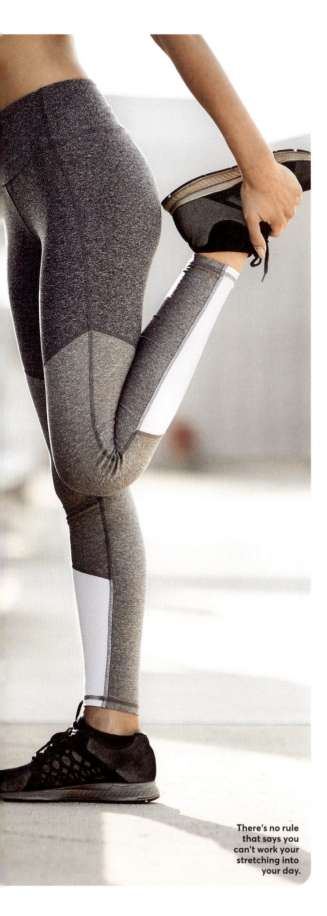

There's no rule that says you can't work your stretching into your day.

8,000

Number of daily steps that significantly reduces mortality risk

Q Will extra exercise help me lose weight?
A Yes. Weight loss is mostly about math. Calories out need to exceed calories in. (Hormonal imbalances can affect this equation, but it's a good place to start.) There's the popular saying, "You can't outrun a bad diet," meaning you need to get your eating under control. Once you have that dialed in, exercise can play a role but it takes effort. The standard exercise guidelines are for health benefits, like helping your heart and lungs to work better and reducing the risk of disease. To lose weight, the ACSM recommends accumulating 300 minutes of aerobic exercise a week or more (if you're doing more vigorous exercise, you can shave some time off that number). And don't forget the weights! In some studies, people who dropped significant pounds and were able to keep them off did an hour of exercise a day.

SLOW WINS THE RACE

▶ Your resting heart rate (RHR)—how fast your ticker runs when you're completely at rest (e.g., in bed)—is a good indicator of your fitness level. Your heart pumps blood throughout your body with each beat; if it can get that job done using fewer beats, it's good for your heart.

Most people's RHR is between 60 and 100, according to the American Heart Association, but 40 to 65 is ideal. Every 10-beat reduction in resting heart rate can translate to a 15 to 20 percent reduction in cardiovascular and all-cause mortality.

Tracking your RHR is a great way to keep an eye on your fitness gains. Take it daily before you get out of bed. It should drop over time as you get fitter. If it starts to increase, it's a sign that you may be overtraining.

6
Exercise Myths Busted!

Are you following workout
theories that are outdated or unsupported?
Let's set the record straight.

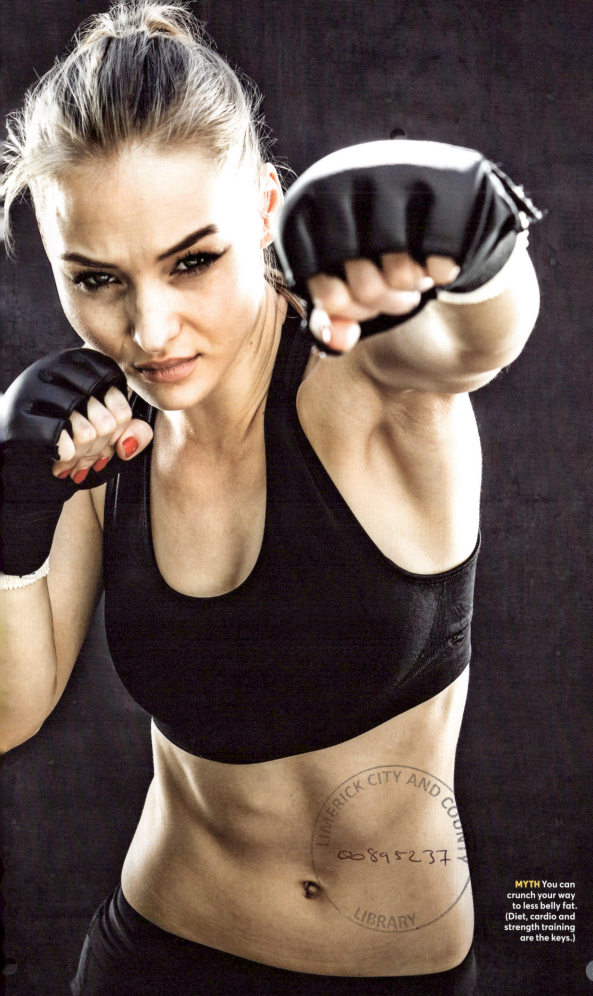

LIMERICK CITY AND COUNTY

00895237

LIBRARY

MYTH You can crunch your way to less belly fat. (Diet, cardio and strength training are the keys.)

21

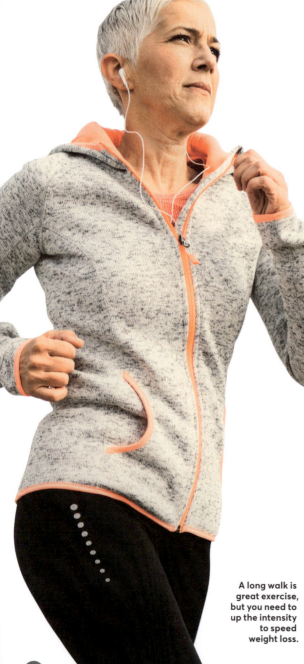

A long walk is great exercise, but you need to up the intensity to speed weight loss.

Given our modern era of "fake news"—and a plethora of fitness "experts"—it's not surprising that so many falsehoods about exercise persist. No matter how many researchers publish good studies debunking these myths, a fair number of people still believe you lose more weight by exercising at a lower intensity or that working out first thing in the morning is far superior to sweating it out any other time of the day. When everything appears so confusing, contradictory or complex, it can seem easier to not even bother working out.

But don't despair. With the help of *real* fitness experts and scientific research, we've busted six common exercise myths. With these facts, you can be more confident about your workouts and get fitter faster.

MYTH NO. 1
You should exercise in the fat-burning zone if you want to lose weight.

Your body taps into different primary sources of energy when you exercise at different heart rates. During higher-intensity workouts, your body burns more carbohydrates than fat, and during lower-intensity workouts, it burns more fat than carbs. So if you're trying to shed pounds, some say it's best to work out in the "fat-burning zone."

First, this zone isn't the same for everyone. A 2009 study found that there's too much variability among individuals to accurately calculate a fat-burning zone outside of a lab setting. And if you ask several fitness experts, each will identify different target heart rates (such as 50 to 65 percent, or 70 to 80 percent of your maximum heart rate) as the fat-burning zone.

Second, even if you could properly gauge your "fat-burning zone" on your own, weight loss comes down to burning more calories (and eating fewer as well). Compared to easier workouts, higher-intensity exercise torches more calories both during and after as your body recovers. You may even burn more calories in less time. And that's what matters if you're trying to shed pounds, says trainer Chris Gagliardi, CSCS, the scientific education content manager for the American Council on Exercise (ACE). Many studies have shown that people (usually those who are overweight) who do high-intensity interval training (HIIT) burn a similar amount of fat—in less time—than those doing more moderate sessions.

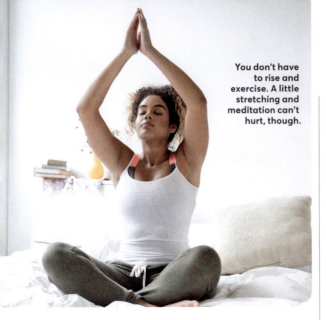

You don't have to rise and exercise. A little stretching and meditation can't hurt, though.

MYTH NO. 2
It's better to exercise in the morning than at other times.

If you're not getting up first thing and sweating, some experts believe you're short-changing yourself. Of course, there are some benefits to this. For one, it pretty much guarantees that you'll get a workout in, rather than getting tied up at work or needing to address a family emergency and never making it to the gym later in the day. For another, some find that starting the day with a good sweat puts them in a great mindset to face whatever arises. Maybe it's because workouts help dampen stress or because that kick-butt kickboxing class makes you feel like nothing can stop you, not even your overflowing inbox.

However, there's no single "best" time to exercise. A research analysis of 11 studies, published in *Chronobiology International*, found that people who did resistance training in the morning or evening showed similar increases in strength (although strength tended to be greater in the evening). Another review found different benefits for doing strength training or cardio exercise at various times of the day. In other words, "there's not enough evidence saying you should always work out in the morning," Gagliardi says. "It's about when you're most likely to do it and how you feel afterward." Find what works best for you, which may mean different times on different days.

MYTH NO. 3
Working out on an empty stomach burns more fat.

Some research suggests that doing cardio or resistance training when fasted (like in the morning) may cause your body to turn to fat, rather than carbohydrates, for fuel. However, research has also found no difference in the number of calories burned during fasted versus non-fasted resistance training. So, as with exercising in the fat-burning zone, it may not pay off in terms of the number on the scale.

Additionally, going into your workout hungry may have negative effects, depending on your activity. If you're doing endurance or high-intensity training, your performance may suffer (in which case you'll *definitely* burn fewer calories). Some experts also theorize that your body may use more protein for fuel in this condition, which leaves less protein to repair and build muscle tissue after your workout.

It's fairly common sense, but experts suggest that if you're doing a shorter, less-intense workout and feel fine without eating for four or more hours beforehand, do so. But if you're going for a long run or a HIIT class, the risk of bonking—and therefore missing out on the maximum strength-gaining and calorie-burning benefits—is probably not worth it. (For more on fueling up the right way pre- and post-workout, see page 38.)

50%
The percentage of exercisers in one recent study who reported working out in the morning. More than a quarter said they opted for evening workouts.

MYTH NO. 4
You can't get strong doing high reps with low weight.

Performing more repetitions with lighter weights is usually associated with increasing muscle endurance. But it can also lead to strength gains when done properly. In a 2016 study published in the *Journal of Applied Physiology*, researchers split 49 men who had experience with weight training into two groups. For 12 weeks, they trained four days a week doing the same exercises. The high-rep group did three sets of 20 to 25 reps using 30 to 50 percent of their one-rep max, while the low-rep group did three sets of eight to 12 reps using 75 to 90 percent of their one-rep max. (Your one-rep max is the heaviest weight you can lift to do a single repetition of an exercise.) At the end of the study, both groups increased lean muscle mass and strength.

Other studies on untrained men found the same thing: A high-rep, low-weight training program leads to similar muscle gains as a low-rep, high-weight protocol. The secret: Lifting to failure, Gagliardi says. Every set, keep doing reps until you truly cannot do one more with good form.

> ## To pick the best time to exercise, think about when you're most likely to do it and how you feel when you're done."
> **—TRAINER CHRIS GAGLIARDI**

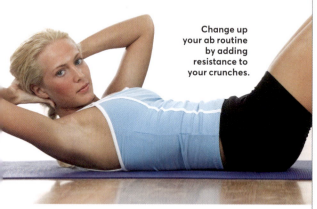

Change up your ab routine by adding resistance to your crunches.

MYTH NO. 5
You should work your abs every day.

Yes, your abs are important, in part because they help with both stability and mobility. But they're like any muscle. "Do you work your legs every day? No, you take two to three days to recover between workouts so you have

better results," says New York City–based health and wellness expert Mike Clancy, CSCS. You should also take time off between ab sessions. Even if your goal is a six-pack, "abs are not developed just by working your abs," Clancy says. "If your goal is muscle definition, that comes from fat loss, and fat loss comes from an energy deficit."

That said, since your entire core (abs, back and glutes) stabilizes the body, doing almost any activity uses them to some extent. But if you're doing actual ab-specific exercises, it's best to hit them no more than three nonconsecutive days a week.

MYTH NO. 6
"Muscle confusion" gives you a better workout.

The theory of "muscle confusion" is that mixing up your workouts from day to day keeps your body guessing, otherwise your muscles adapt to the exercises and your efforts to build muscle or lose fat will plateau. But the research on this concept is mixed.

It appears that it's best to have at least *some* structure to a fitness program. For example, in a 2014 study published in the *Journal of Strength and Conditioning Research*, men followed one of five training programs: varied exercises of constant intensity; varied exercises of varied intensity; constant exercises of constant intensity; constant exercises of varied intensity; or a control plan. After 12 weeks, the men who did varied exercises at constant intensity had greater strength gains compared to the others.

Similarly, in another study of 21 men published in *PLOS ONE* in 2019, the "muscle confusion" group actually followed a strategic plan: The "randomly chosen" exercises that they performed during each upper- and lower-body workout were selected to evenly target their muscles so that they worked both the fronts and backs of their bodies. Compared to another group who did the same exercises each workout, but who increased their intensity over time, this "randomized" group made similar gains in strength after eight weeks, but were more motivated to train.

So the biggest benefit of muscle confusion may be that the novelty keeps you interested, so you stick with it. "You need strategic adjustment to exercise," Clancy says. Exercises are a bit like skills for the body to learn. Doing them with a plan that allows you to perfect the movement and then gradually add load will boost performance and strength.

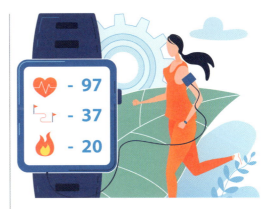

WHAT CAN 10 MINUTES DO FOR YOU?

▶ The U.S. Physical Activity Guidelines recommend aiming for about 30 minutes of moderate physical activity every day. You may have heard that if you can't fit in 30 minutes all at once, try doing three 10-minute bouts throughout the day. But can 10 minutes of exercise really make a difference? It sure can. In an analysis published in *Sports Medicine* in 2019, researchers reviewed 19 studies involving more than 1,000 adults. These studies compared the effects of one workout with those of multiple shorter workouts that used the same type of exercise and intensity and added up to the same total amount of sweat time. In the end, there was no difference in the participants' level of fitness, blood pressure, lipids (cholesterol), insulin and glucose. "Collectively, our findings suggest that adults are likely to accrue similar health benefits from exercising in a single bout or accumulating activity from shorter bouts throughout the day," the study's authors conclude. In fact, according to the U.S. Department of Health and Human Services, "moderate-to-vigorous physical activity of *any* duration counts toward meeting the key guidelines."

▶ Just keep in mind what your goals are. If you're currently pretty sedentary, 10 minutes is fantastic. "Research shows that if you do any amount of physical activity above what you normally do, there can be health-related benefits," Chris Gagliardi, CSCS, says. If, say, you're training for a race, you'll need to work up to longer runs. And if your goal is muscle growth, you'll need to do multiple reps and sets in one workout to fatigue the muscles, he says.

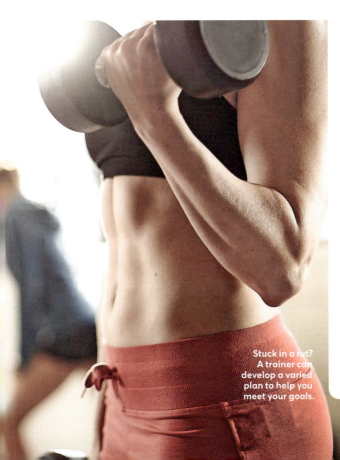

Stuck in a rut? A trainer can develop a varied plan to help you meet your goals.

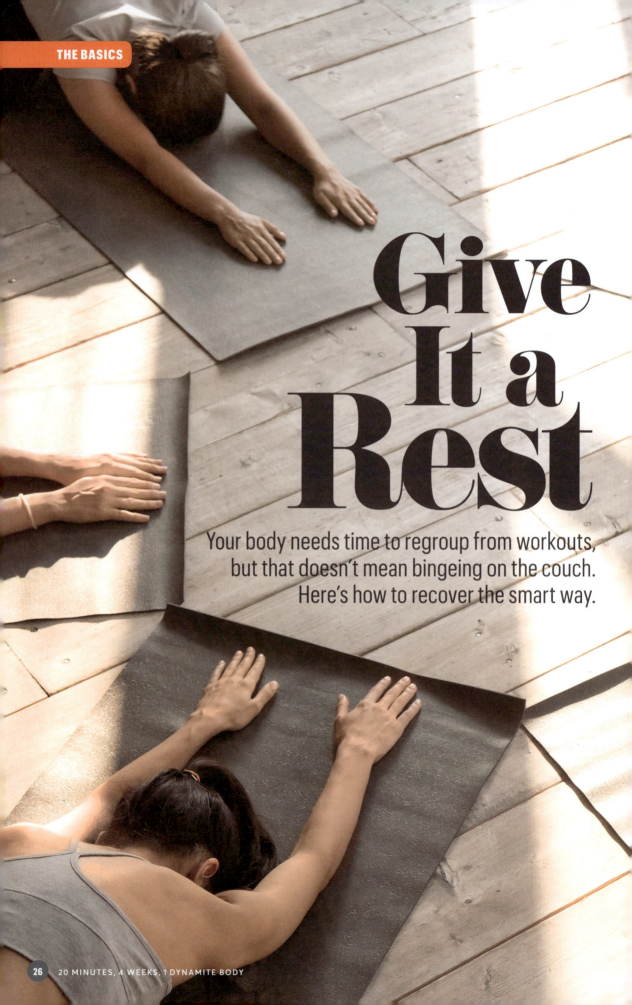

Give It a Rest

Your body needs time to regroup from workouts, but that doesn't mean bingeing on the couch. Here's how to recover the smart way.

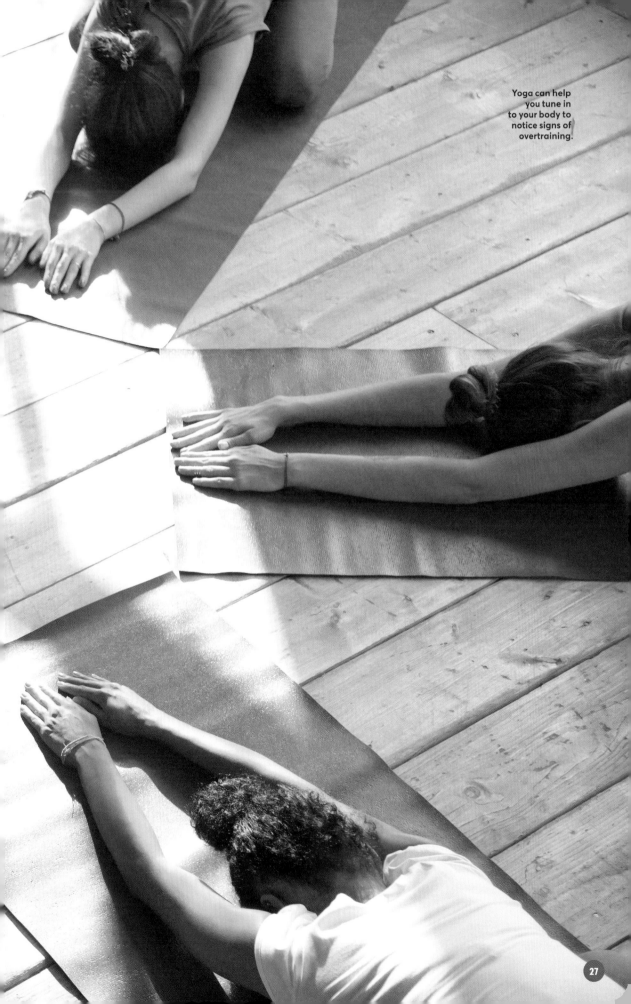

Yoga can help
you tune in
to your body to
notice signs of
overtraining.

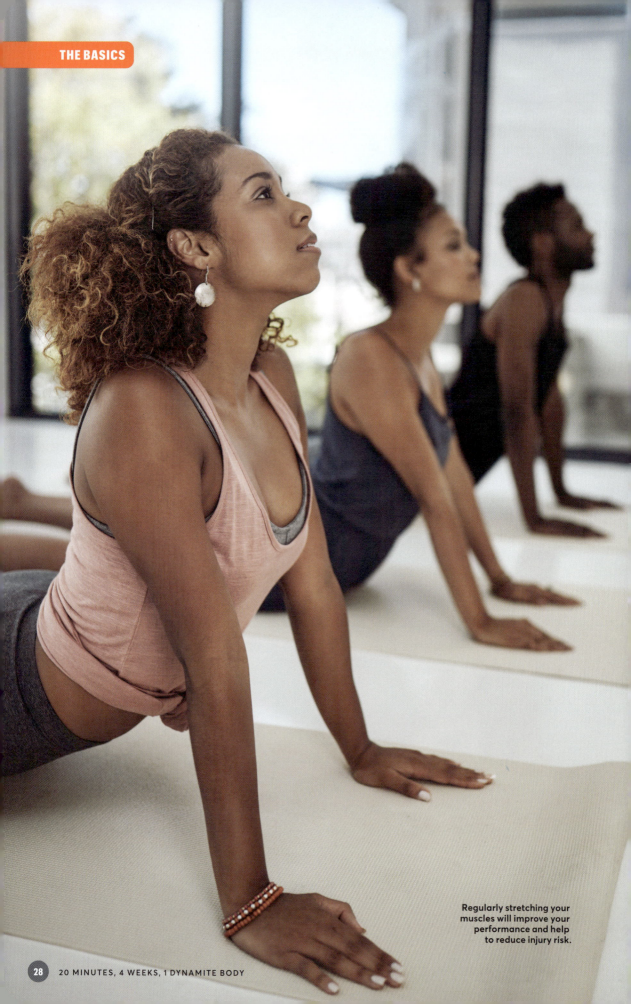

Regularly stretching your muscles will improve your performance and help to reduce injury risk.

O f all the hot trends in fitness today—from HIIT to indoor cycling to streaming workouts —there's one that's especially surprising: doing less. Taking a note from athletes' playbooks, everyday fitness enthusiasts are embracing rest days as a way to give both muscles and mind a break, as well as to boost performance, guard against injury and, ultimately, grow stronger.

"I've found that most people still don't take enough rest days, but yes, it's a growing movement," says Kevin Kilkenny, ATC, an athletic trainer who has worked with the New York Jets, and who co-owns Generations Physical Therapy in West Islip, New York. Recovery, he says, "is just giving the body a chance to replenish and heal again from the workout you've had. It also prevents wear and tear and strain on joints, tendonitis and other injuries that would come from overdoing it."

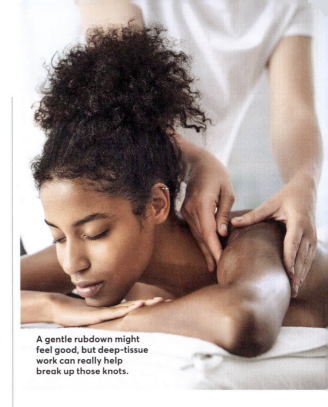

A gentle rubdown might feel good, but deep-tissue work can really help break up those knots.

A Time to Build

You may think that exercise is what builds muscles, but that's actually when they get broken down, says Josh Yellen, ATC, EdD, director of the Master of Athletic Training Program at the University of Houston. When greater-than-usual resistance is placed on muscles due to activities like weightlifting and intense cardio exercise, microscopic tears occur in their fibers, explains Kilkenny. The strengthening really happens on the rest day: "When the body repairs these tears, it pulls those fibers back in, making them stronger and more taut," he says.

The alternative—to keep hitting your workout hard every day—can create real problems. "As we push, and we push, and we push, little injuries that may arise can become very big injuries pretty quickly," Yellen explains. Even if you don't end up injured, your results will start to be compromised, too.

"If you're not resting enough, then the muscle is not fully recovered and when you start working it again, that causes it to tighten up and shorten in length and you end up developing muscle fatigue and tightness earlier," says Kilkenny. "If you're starting to

feel run-down, and you're not getting the good workout that you normally do, usually that's when your body's saying, 'Hey, I need to take a break.' The muscles will get stronger and healthier with the correct recovery."

Two Types of Taking It Easy

The very word "rest" probably brings up a delicious image of sitting on the sofa with the remote control at your elbow. Not so fast. When it comes to rest days, there are two types: active and passive. Knowing the difference is key, since the right kind of recovery—usually an active one—will help you get over your post-workout discomfort and prepare for your next session more quickly.

"Active recovery starts right after exercise, during the cool-down," says Kilkenny. "It also means doing dynamic [movement-based vs. static holding] stretching, massage and yoga the day after a tough session (and maybe even 48 hours later if you're still sore). During active rest, you might even work the same muscles you did during your tough session but in a less intense way. Say you did a killer group-cycling class with a ton of hills, and the next day you can't walk up the stairs. The best thing to do is light exercise, whether it's taking an easy bike ride, walking or doing yoga. Those activities will help break down the lactic acid [an acid that accumulates in

Foam rollers help get at muscle adhesions and provide a sense of "ah" for especially tight areas.

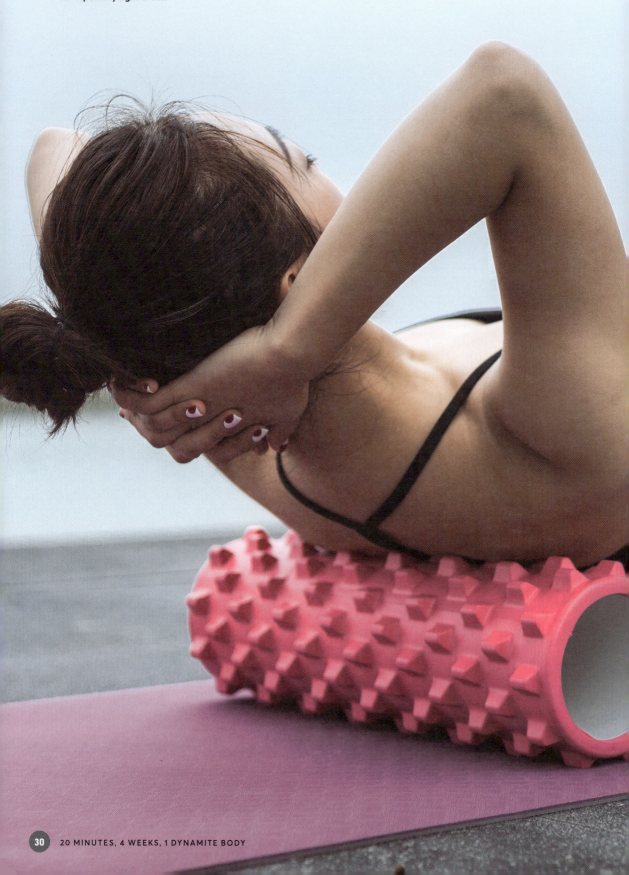

SIX WAYS TO REDUCE POST-WORKOUT MUSCLE SORENESS

Soreness and exercise sometimes go hand in hand. But there are scientifically proven ways to reduce the discomfort.

▶ **GET A MASSAGE** Recent studies have shown that a post-workout massage reduces delayed-onset muscle soreness (DOMS) as well as blood markers for inflammation and tissue damage. It can also reduce how fatigued you feel.

▶ **TRY FOAM ROLLING** Both foam rolling (with those long round tubes) and massage provide myofascial release, which means they alleviate tension and adhesions (knots) in the connective tissue of your muscles. One small study, published in the *Journal of Athletic Training*, found that using a foam roller after exercise helped alleviate muscle fatigue and DOMS, as well as improve muscular performance.

▶ **DRINK TART CHERRY JUICE** Strange but true: A Scandinavian study of recreational marathon runners found that those who drank tart cherry juice before, during and after their runs recovered their muscle strength significantly faster. In part, this is because substances in the juice reduce muscle inflammation.

▶ **HAVE A COUPLE OF CUPS OF COFFEE** A study published in the *Journal of Pain* found that when people had the equivalent of about two cups of brewed coffee an hour before their workout, the incidence of DOMS decreased by nearly 50 percent.

▶ **SPIN AFTER A TOUGH WORKOUT** One study of women found that those who cycled at low or medium intensity for 20 minutes after a workout designed to induce DOMS had both a reduction in muscle pain and a boost in muscle strength.

▶ **SNACK ON SOME SALMON** A study in the *Clinical Journal of Sport Medicine* found that people who took omega-3's, an essential fatty acid that can help fight inflammation, had less self-perceived pain and a greater range of motion at 48 hours post-exercise. (Foods rich in omega-3s include salmon, sardines and other fatty fish; flax; chia seeds; and walnuts.)

the muscles during exercise and can make you sore and fatigued] that has built up."

By contrast, passive recovery is when you don't do anything exercise-related beyond your normal activities of daily living. "We rely on passive rest more in overuse injuries, when we're like, 'Look, you need to take a day or two off and do nothing. Your body just needs to heal,'" says Yellen. He admits that for some people, these days are very hard: "They feel like they need to do *something*," he says. Reserve passive rest days for when you're experiencing symptoms beyond soreness. "You're looking at your overall body fatigue, sleep and how you're dealing with stress," says Yellen. If you have problems in any of these areas, it's time to take a break.

Rest Done Right

It would be great if there were hard-and-fast rules about when to rest, but Kilkenny and Yellen agree that it varies from person to person and depends on how you're training.

"A lot of times, even that first day after you work out is not so bad," he explains. Most people aren't going to feel soreness until 24 to 72 hours after a workout." This phenomenon is known as delayed-onset muscle soreness, aka DOMS. "It's the *second* day after that you hear people saying, 'Oh my god, I can't move.' That's when you need to take another active rest day, even if you just took one the day before." You'll know it's time to return to your workout when the soreness is about 80 percent gone, he adds.

Most savvy and experienced athletes, Kilkenny says, "will have recovery days built in. They try to go four days with an off day, then three days and another off day." On their "on" days, "they mix it up and don't do the same thing each time," Kilkenny says. "That's when the overuse injuries come in." Unless you're training for a specific competition, most people can get away with taking one passive or active rest day a week. When you start to get that tired, uninspired feeling, then take a full day off, with no guilt.

Recovery is "all about listening to your body," Yellen explains. Tune in to its messages, and you'll get better results.

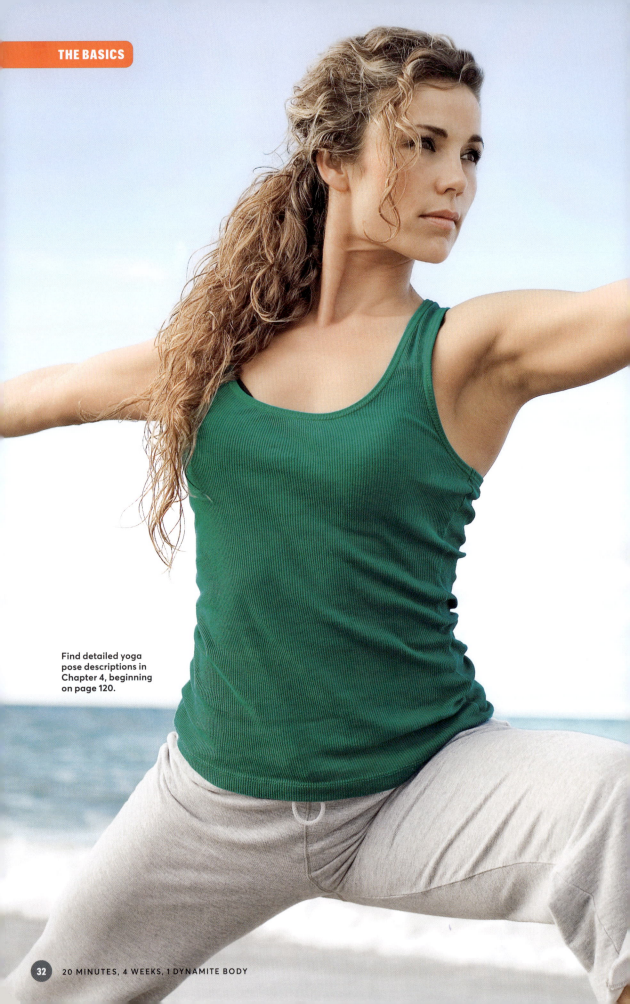

Find detailed yoga pose descriptions in Chapter 4, beginning on page 120.

Find Your Way Om

Feed your heart, mind and muscles by choosing the type of yoga that meets your total health goals.

Many exercisers initially flock to yoga for the physical benefits, including enhanced flexibility, strength and balance and a stronger core. Others come to it as a much-needed way to slow down (physically and mentally) and chill out. "Yogis often start a new practice to work out an injury that's sidelined their regular workouts or reduce the effects of stress," says Ellen Barrett, author of *Yogini Workout* and star of 50-plus workouts on ellenbarrett.com.

These seemingly simple benefits have very real effects on health, too. Research from the American Osteopathic Association, in fact, shows that relaxation techniques—like deep breathing and yoga—can lessen chronic pain, arthritis discomfort, insomnia and headaches. A study published in the journal *Spine* found that people with back pain who performed two 90-minute yoga sessions a week for 24 weeks experienced a 56 percent reduction in chronic pain on average.

This is when you start to realize there's so much more to this ancient practice than just holding a pose for a few breaths. The yoga poses were created as a way to quiet the body in preparation for long, seated meditations, which the original yogis viewed as the really important work of yoga. Many studies have explored the practice's calming effect—even just 20 minutes of asana, or poses, a day can make a difference—on brain chemicals (aka neurotransmitters), making it an excellent remedy for depression and anxiety. The breath work and mindfulness aspects of yoga may be the practice's superpowers. They help balance the sympathetic (fight or flight) and parasympathetic (rest and digest) nervous systems in a way that movement alone can't.

I'm In! Now What?

Ready to embrace your inner lotus flower? It may take some experimenting to find the right class for you. While you can practice in a studio, online or just by yourself, if you're a newbie, it's best to start with an instructor who can walk you through the process, correct your form and deepen your understanding of some of the principles. (Many studios offer freebies for first-timers.) "I didn't know what to expect. I started yoga and then I stopped. Then I started again," says instructor Kelly DiNardo, RYT, owner of Past Tense yoga studio in Washington, D.C. "I did years of yoga on and off until I found the athletic, flowing vinyasa style of yoga that resonates with me."

You can find certified instructors through Yoga Alliance (yogaalliance.org), and DiNardo recommends bringing a friend to class to bolster your confidence. Once you get a handle on how it works, you can take advantage of all the great yoga apps and streaming workouts that are available, such as Glo and Gaia.

What's Your Yoga Style?

There are many different styles of asanas, and the only way to figure out which one is right for you is to try them. Each will include an emphasis on soothing breath, postures and mindfulness, which they incorporate in different ways.

ASHTANGA This is a flowing, very athletic style of class, but ashtanga devotees perform poses in a strict order each time. There are six series, each of which includes more than a dozen poses, and you'll usually only get through a portion during a class, especially as a beginner. The goal is to memorize the series so you can move through them on your own at home.

HOT YOGA At 85 F and climbing, yoga in a heated room is designed to enhance your natural flexibility and initiate sweating to help purify the body. Some classes perform a set series of moves, while others are less rigid. Look for Hot 8 Yoga, Baptiste Yoga and CorePower Yoga.

IYENGAR Super-precise Iyengar instructors introduce blocks and straps to slowly ease you into perfect alignment, and keep you there, making it ideal for beginners and purists. There's an emphasis on controlled movements and learning how to hold a pose calmly. Some participants claim that certain postures almost feel like physical therapy stretches.

KUNDALINI You remain on the floor with seated twists and supine postures that favor faster repetitions—think 60 leg lifts, yoga-style. But kundalini also offers long meditations, chanting and, very often, live music. Each style of yoga provides a different way to connect with the ancient wisdom of yoga, and this is one of the most spiritual practices around.

YIN YOGA A soothing and restorative practice, yin stretches and strengthens connective tissue (muscles, tendons and ligaments) during poses that are held for two to five minutes. You'll use props—straps, blocks and bolsters—to make it easier to release into each pose, and part of the goal is to train your brain to relax into the stretch as well. It's not always as easy and relaxing as it sounds!

15 MORE REASONS TO TRY YOGA

According to Harvard Medical School, the scientific community is barely scratching the surface of what yoga can potentially do for health. According to research, it:

▶ Boosts athletic performance
▶ Revs metabolism
▶ Improves heart health
▶ Decreases resting heart rate
▶ Soothes menopause symptoms
▶ Eases carpal tunnel syndrome
▶ Increases mental clarity
▶ Cultivates emotional healing
▶ Improves posture
▶ Hones balance
▶ Decreases stress hormones
▶ Aids digestion
▶ Eases symptoms of irritable bowel syndrome
▶ Increases bone density in the spine
▶ Lowers blood sugar and "bad" cholesterol

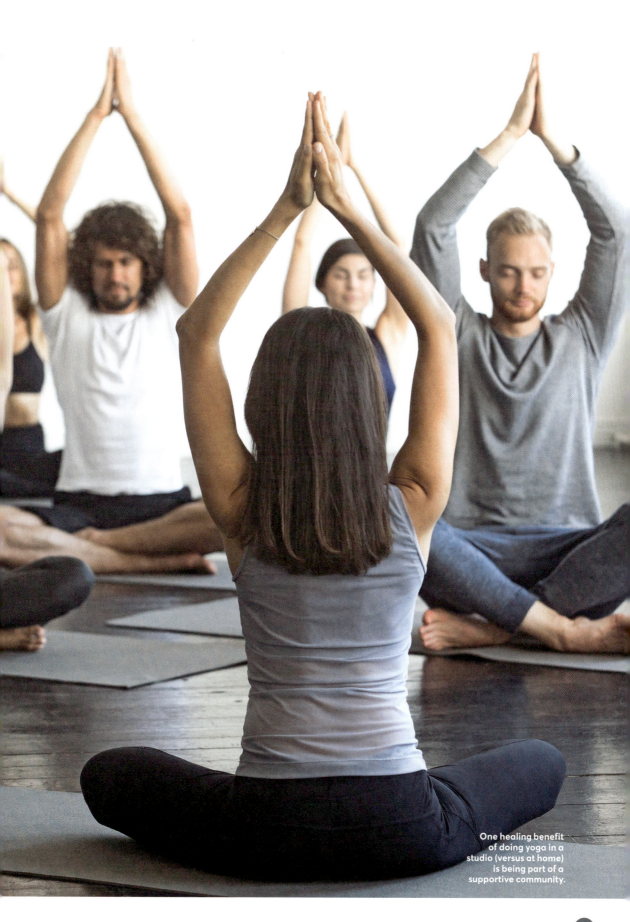

One healing benefit
of doing yoga in a
studio (versus at home)
is being part of a
supportive community.

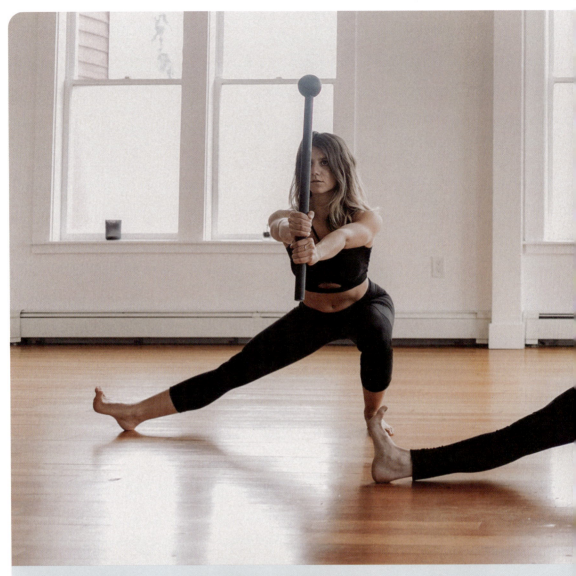

HYBRID YOGA WORKOUTS

Combining asanas with another type of exercise adds variety to your weekly routine, plus it's time efficient. "Popular Pi-Yo classes have always interwoven Sun Salutations with standing and seated Pilates core work," says yoga and Pilates instructor Ellen Barrett. You can also find yoga mixed with weights, cycling, dance, farm animals, weed and more. Check out these two-for-one workouts to add oomph to your practice.

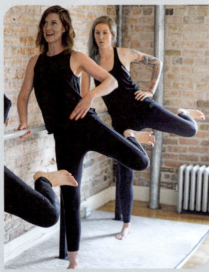

◄YOGA BARRE

You'll never have to choose between a ballet class and a yoga session again. At both Hot Yoga Barre studios in Richmond, Virginia, teachers turn up the burn with high-intensity Sun Salutations and innumerable leg lifts at the barre. You may use exercise bands and other sculpting tools, too. (You can find similar classes around the country, or check out thehotyogabarre.com.)

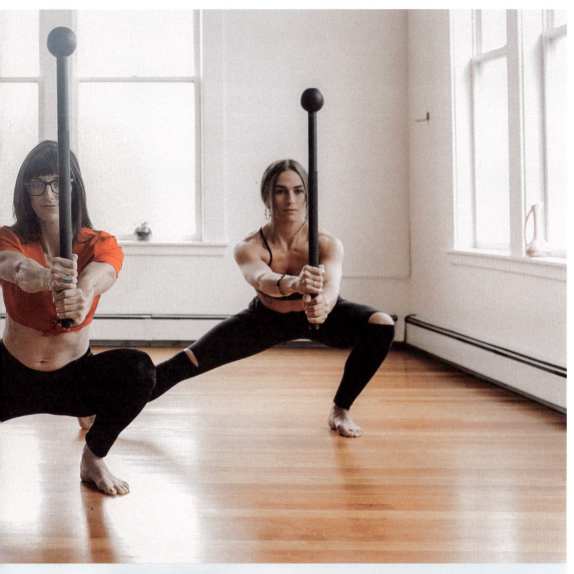

▲ **STEEL MACE VINYASA** Taking the yoga-with-dumbbells idea a *big* step further, creator Summer Huntington uses 5- and 7-pound maces in her flowing yoga classes. The movement combined with the unwieldy weight is a recipe for serious sweating and strengthening. Find Huntington's virtual classes at steelmacevinyasa.com.

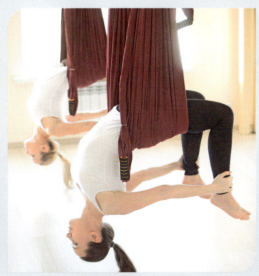

◀ **AERIAL YOGA** Explore your inner Cirque du Soleil performer by draping yourself in a soft silk or rayon "hammock" or swing. The rigging helps develop core strength, flexibility and spine stability as you move. (It beats ab crunches by a mile.) Inversions (upside-down poses) become easier and more relaxing and Yin classes are simply dreamy in the silks. Classes are offered in studios throughout the U.S., find some listings at antigravityfitness.com for places near you.

Fuel Up

The right food at the right time will give you the energy you need to crush every sweat session.

You won't get too far on an empty gas tank, and the same goes for your workouts. "If you don't eat enough, your body won't have the fuel to power through," says Jim White, RDN, owner of Jim White Fitness and Nutrition Studios. "Your body needs protein for muscle synthesis and carbohydrates for glycogen storage."

Luckily, for the average person who's not training for an event or sport, it's not too hard to stay on track. As long as you eat a balanced meal or snack (something with carbs, protein and maybe a little fat) about one to four hours pre-workout and again about two hours post-workout, you should be good.

It goes without saying (almost) that—like gasoline in your valuable automobile—the better-quality fuel you put in your body, the better performance you can expect. Whether it's pre- or post-workout, load up on vegetables and fruit, whole grains and legumes, lean, high-quality protein (minimal hormones and antibiotics) and healthy fat. Here's how to do it:

WHAT TO EAT BEFOREHAND

CARBOHYDRATES

Yes, carbs are your main source of quick energy for exercise. However, in most cases you don't need to obsess over downing something right before a workout as long as you've eaten a meal or snack that contains nutritious (not junk food) carbs one to four hours before exercising. And morning exercisers are probably fine hitting it on an empty stomach, depending on the length and intensity of your session.

"For moderate-intensity cardio workouts, you don't need carbohydrates immediately before," says nutrition consultant Mike Roussell, PhD. But if you run for longer than an hour, you will need some carbs during your session to keep your glycogen stores (read: your muscles' fuel) stocked.

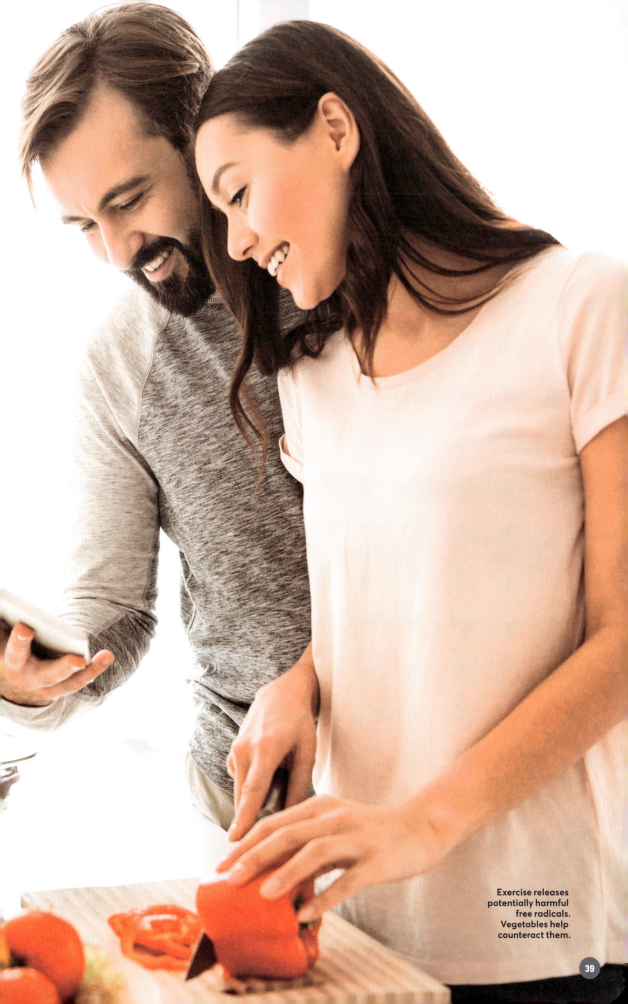

Exercise releases potentially harmful free radicals. Vegetables help counteract them.

And while high-intensity workouts like HIIT burn more carbohydrates than less-intense programs, they're also usually short. "Your body has ample stored carbohydrates in your muscles to meet the needs of these workouts," says Roussell. That's if you're eating regular meals and not restricting calories in a significant way. At the same time, though, eating some carbs before doing HIIT can make those burpees *feel* a little easier mentally, he adds. If you find yourself struggling, physically or mentally, have a snack before your next workout to see how it changes things.

Haven't eaten in four hours? Consume 15 to 30 grams of easily digestible carbs about a half hour before you exercise. That might be a banana or a sports drink; both provide fast energy and are easy on your stomach.

PROTEIN

"Pre-workout protein has not been shown to have a significant benefit with weight training," Roussell says. But if you have protein from solid food sources—not a drink—about

60 to 90 minutes before your workout, that protein will help with your *post*-workout recovery. "The amino acids will peak in your bloodstream at the right time," he explains.

This is particularly important if you're trying to increase muscle size or strength. White recommends consuming at least 20 to 30 grams of lean protein before a strength session. Try eggs, chicken breast, fish, soy, quinoa or pistachios. (Protein drinks are digested too quickly, so they won't help you post-workout.)

FATS

Too much fat can slow digestion and lead to gastrointestinal distress during a workout. Aim to eat less than 10 grams of healthy fats—such as nuts, nut butter, seeds or avocado—in your pre-workout meal or snack, White says.

WHAT TO EAT AFTERWARD

CARBOHYDRATES

"A limited number of people—mostly those competing at an elite level—need to concern

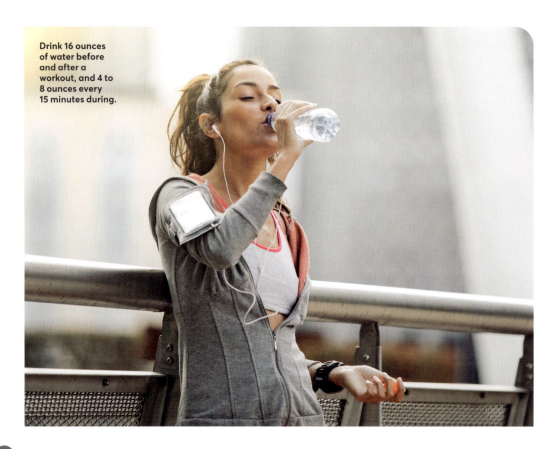

Drink 16 ounces of water before and after a workout, and 4 to 8 ounces every 15 minutes during.

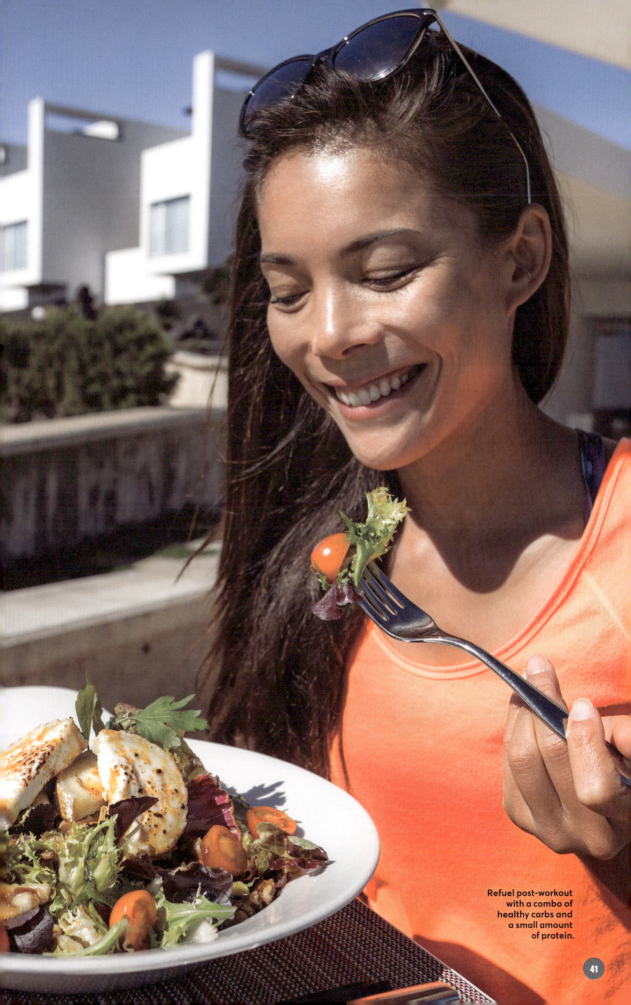

Refuel post-workout
with a combo of
healthy carbs and
a small amount
of protein.

themselves with immediate replenishment of muscle glycogen stores," Roussell says. Everyone else won't completely empty their glycogen supplies during a workout and will eat enough before their next session to refill them. "By replenishing your muscle glycogen over time with the carbohydrates in your meals, you have the freedom to eat your calories versus feeling like you have to drink them right after exercise," Roussell says.

To make sure you're restocking the right way, choose complex carbs, such as oatmeal, sweet or white potatoes, brown rice, whole-wheat bread or pasta or quinoa at meals.

PROTEIN

"A small amount of protein paired with carbs provides amino acids to help reduce inflammation and repair and build muscle tissue," White explains. In a meta-analysis of 23 studies published in the *Journal of the International Society of Sports Nutrition*, researchers found no association between protein timing and muscle growth. What did matter was how much protein the study subjects consumed throughout the day.

"Having protein within 90 minutes of your workout is ideal to stop muscle breakdown and also to help maximize your body's ability to build and repair muscle," Roussell says. But, White adds, "the regular meals you consume following exercise are also important for muscle growth." So if you're strength training and can fit in a meal or snack with 25 to 30 grams of protein in those 90 minutes, great. If not, be sure to eat meals that each contain that much protein throughout the day. Choose lean options like whey or pea protein shakes (look for a product that contains 3 grams of the amino acid leucine per serving to maximize muscle building), lean meats, eggs, unsweetened Greek yogurt, cottage cheese and peanut butter.

FATS

They're not necessary post-workout. Plus, high-fat meals "could slow the uptake and digestion of the protein and carbs that you want to get into your system as quickly as possible" post-workout if you're an athlete, Roussell explains.

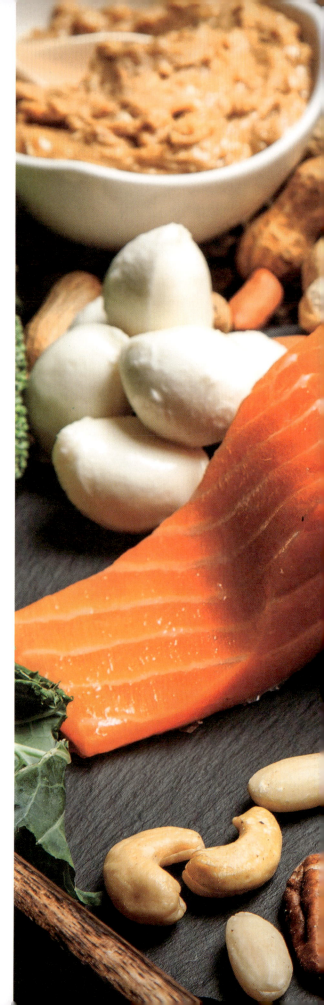

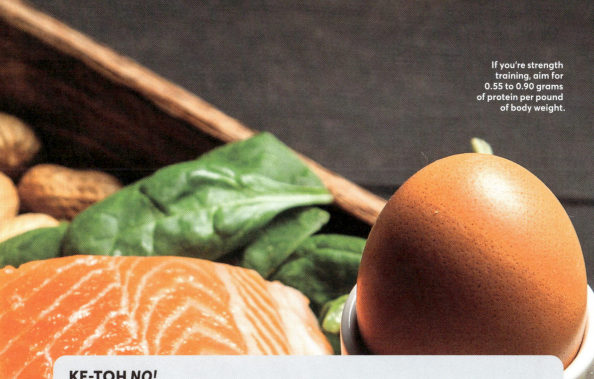

If you're strength training, aim for 0.55 to 0.90 grams of protein per pound of body weight.

KE-TOH *NO!*

Is your trendy diet undermining your fitness goals? Fueling up before a workout and replenishing your body afterward is pretty straightforward if you eat a variety of foods and macronutrients (fat, protein and carbohydrates). But things can be harder if you're following a nutrition plan that restricts certain macronutrients, which many of them do. Here's what dietitians say to be mindful of if you try some of the hottest eating styles.

THE DIET Intermittent fasting
HOW IT CAN HURT If you're doing a low-intensity workout while fasting, you should be fine. "But for high-intensity workouts [if you've been fasting], I recommend eating carbs beforehand because you need energy," says Jim White, RDN, owner of Jim White Fitness and Nutrition Studios. Otherwise you might bonk or simply not be able to work out as hard as you want.
THE FIX Do your workouts (strength or more-demanding cardio) midday or later so that you have something in your stomach.

THE DIET Paleo
HOW IT CAN HURT Some Paleo plans are stricter than others, and different plans also recommend varying amounts of protein, fats and carbs. If you follow a super-low-carb Paleo diet, you risk not having adequate fuel for your workouts.
THE FIX Consider cycling your carbs. Follow the low-carb guidelines on days you don't work out, and on days you do exercise, up your intake and consume carbs before and after your session.

THE DIET Ketogenic
HOW IT CAN HURT Same as with Paleo: "Going low-carb can decrease your energy; you might hit a wall and not be able to get through your workout," White says.
THE FIX Your body should adapt to using fat as a primary fuel source after about six to eight weeks, says nutrition consultant Mike Roussell, PhD. During those first months, "don't cut calories too much," he says. "Being hypocaloric and having your body adapt to a new fuel source is making it hard on yourself for no reason." Also skew toward less-intense aerobic exercise.

THE DIET Vegan
HOW IT CAN HURT Those athletes in the documentary *The Game Changers*? They all have trainers and many have chefs and nutritionists so they're sure to get all the protein they need to build muscle. The average person trying to follow a vegan diet, however, could fall short on protein as well as calcium, which plays a role in muscle contraction and therefore growth, White explains. That shortchanges results.
THE FIX If you're trying to eat vegan, make higher-protein plant foods such as tempeh, seitan, lentils, tofu and beans staples in your diet, and also consume a protein shake. "It's really hard to get those protein numbers up to the recommended amount for muscle building," White says. Then, in addition to drinking fortified plant-based milks, consider taking a calcium-vitamin D supplement.

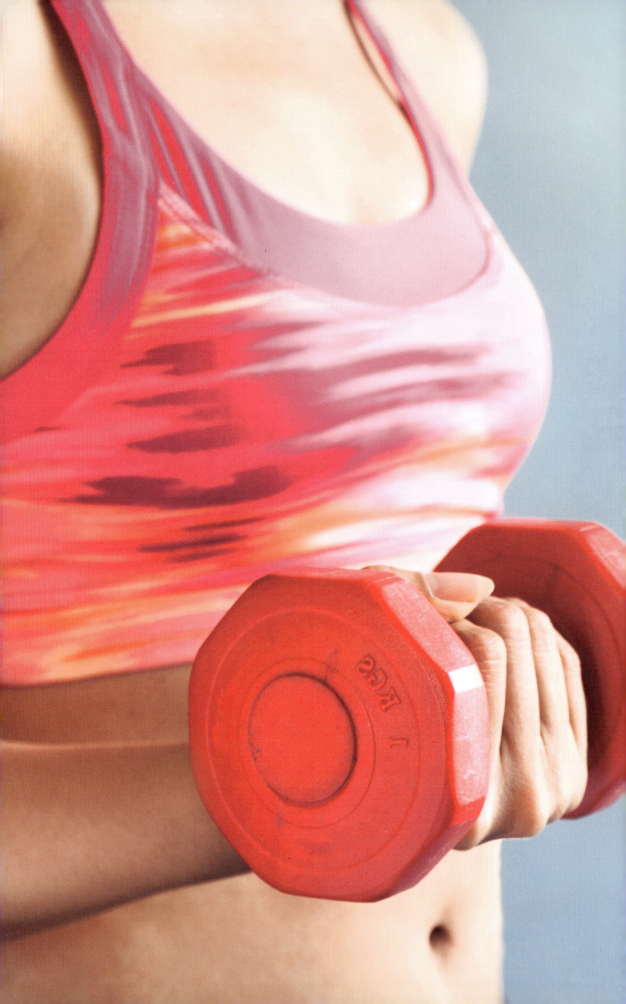

GAINING STRENGTH

↓

Get Firm & Lean

RESISTANCE TRAINING BUILDS MUSCLE, KEEPS YOUR METABOLISM STOKED AND CAN HELP YOU STAVE OFF WEIGHT GAIN AS YOU GET OLDER. (AND NO, YOU WON'T GET BULKY!)

Change Gear

Stock your home gym with these tools and you may never need a club membership again.

Y ou don't have to use equipment to work out: Your own body weight is resistance enough for strength moves in many cases. But if you want to keep getting fitter and stronger, a few tools can come in handy. Plus, sometimes working out gets a little boring and having some new equipment to spice things up can keep your brain engaged and provide new ways for your muscles to get stronger. The following items will bring you almost endless ways to stick with your routine—and enjoy it.

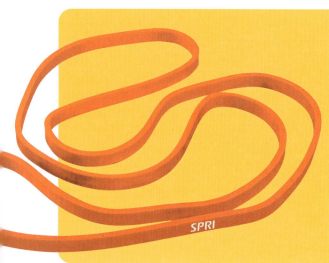

SPRI

Resistance Bands

Extra-thick superbands give your regular resistance-band workouts added heft and provide options for multijoint exercises. Use them for squats, deadlifts, pull-up training, core work and more.

TRY THIS MOVE Step inside the band and place one side around the back of your waist. Cross the band and stand with feet hip-width apart on the other side of the band, so it makes an X in front of your body. (You'll probably have to squat down at least halfway to do this.) Stay in the half squat and step right foot out to right, then bring left foot in so feet are hip-width apart again. Continue, taking 12 steps to the right, then 12 steps back to the left. (For more band exercises, turn to page 84.)

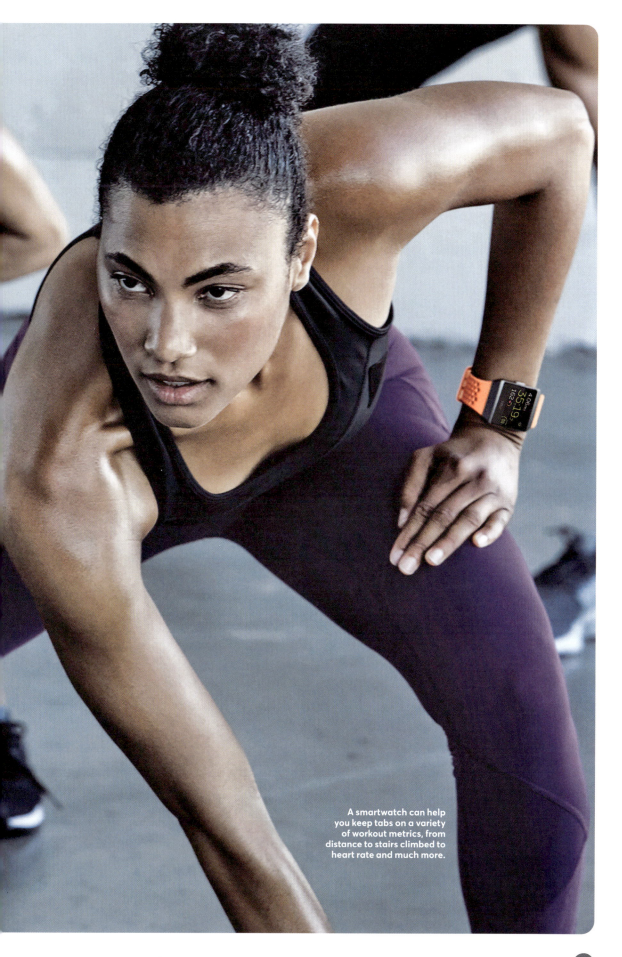

A smartwatch can help you keep tabs on a variety of workout metrics, from distance to stairs climbed to heart rate and much more.

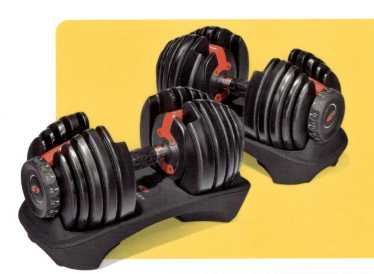

Adjustable Dumbbells

Customizable handweights (like these from Bowflex, which adjust from 5 pounds to 52.5 pounds) mean you don't have to store several pairs in your home gym in order to get a good workout. After all, different muscle groups require different amounts of resistance to get stronger. Look for an adjustable option that has several different settings, and that they can be switched safely and easily.

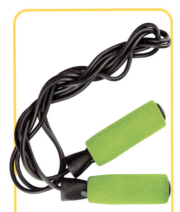

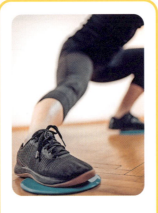

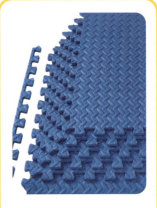

Jump Rope

A jump rope provides built-in cardio that travels with you. Use it on its own or in between moves for a high-intensity boost (you'll burn about 10 calories a minute). For more arm toning and cardiovascular conditioning, opt for a weighted rope.
TRY THIS MOVE Add a jump rope to your burpees for crazy conditioning: Holding the ends of the rope in each hand, swing it overhead to the floor in front of you, then squat, place hands on floor and jump feet back into plank position. Lower body to floor, push back up, jump feet forward and jump up, swinging rope under feet; repeat for 30 to 60 seconds.

Gliding Discs

These simple, paper plate–like contraptions were the first to capitalize on using the resistance of your body weight against the floor. Get them for hardwoods or carpet and use them under your hands or feet for strengthening or quick cardio. (You can use paper plates for the same thing, but these will hold up over time.)
TRY THIS MOVE Stand with feet hip-width apart and right foot on a disc. Squat on left leg as you slide right foot out to side, feet parallel. Slowly draw right leg back in to center and repeat. Do 12 reps then switch legs and repeat to complete one set.

Exercise Mat

Having a little padding under your back makes many floor moves a lot more comfortable, and offers a no-slip surface for standing exercises. Some home gym users prefer to skip thinner yoga mats in favor of foam flooring, like this Exercise Puzzle Mat from ProsourceFit. Models like this feature interlocking tiles that suit your space.
TRY THIS MOVE Lie faceup on the floor, knees bent and feet flat with ankles aligned under knees (legs are hip-width apart). Lift hips so body is straight from knees to chest, then extend right leg toward ceiling. Keep hips level as you pulse up 15 times, squeezing left glute. Switch legs and repeat.

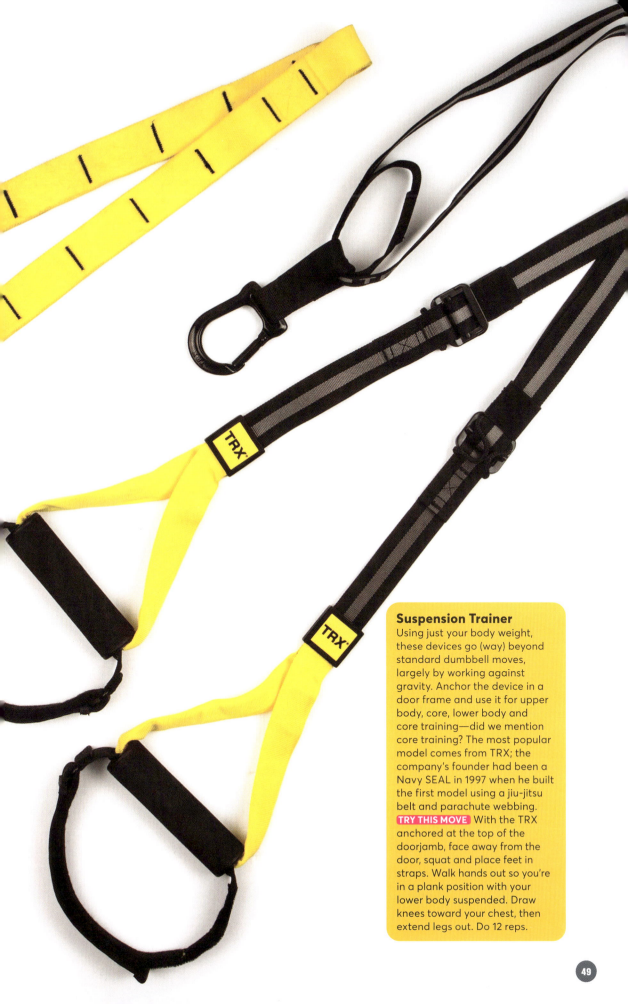

Suspension Trainer

Using just your body weight, these devices go (way) beyond standard dumbbell moves, largely by working against gravity. Anchor the device in a door frame and use it for upper body, core, lower body and core training—did we mention core training? The most popular model comes from TRX; the company's founder had been a Navy SEAL in 1997 when he built the first model using a jiu-jitsu belt and parachute webbing. **TRY THIS MOVE** With the TRX anchored at the top of the doorjamb, face away from the door, squat and place feet in straps. Walk hands out so you're in a plank position with your lower body suspended. Draw knees toward your chest, then extend legs out. Do 12 reps.

Strong From Head to Toe

This high-energy routine hits every muscle, including your heart.

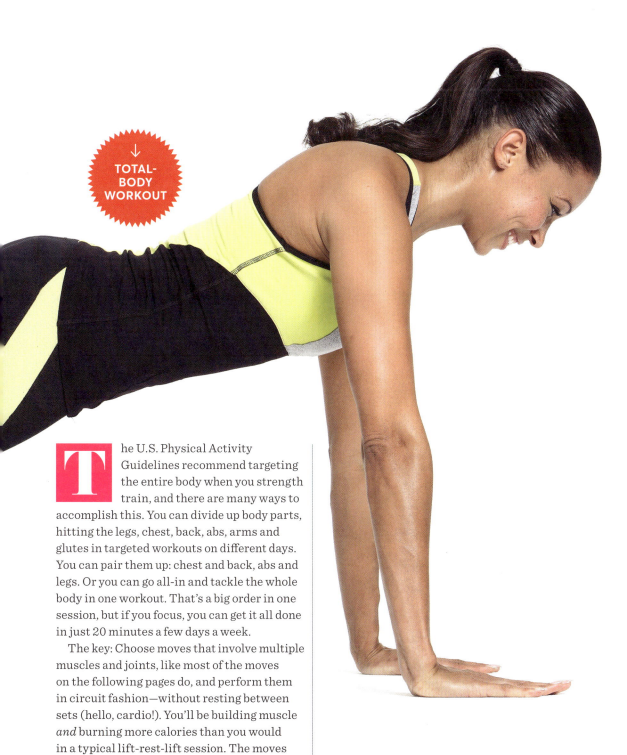

↓
TOTAL-BODY WORKOUT

The U.S. Physical Activity Guidelines recommend targeting the entire body when you strength train, and there are many ways to accomplish this. You can divide up body parts, hitting the legs, chest, back, abs, arms and glutes in targeted workouts on different days. You can pair them up: chest and back, abs and legs. Or you can go all-in and tackle the whole body in one workout. That's a big order in one session, but if you focus, you can get it all done in just 20 minutes a few days a week.

The key: Choose moves that involve multiple muscles and joints, like most of the moves on the following pages do, and perform them in circuit fashion—without resting between sets (hello, cardio!). You'll be building muscle *and* burning more calories than you would in a typical lift-rest-lift session. The moves here include higher-energy exercises that use large muscles (they guzzle more calories when you use them) as well as some more focused exercises that require precision—no autopilot lifting allowed here. Ready, set, sculpt!

Push-up tip: Squeeze your glutes and engage your abs before you start to bend your arms.

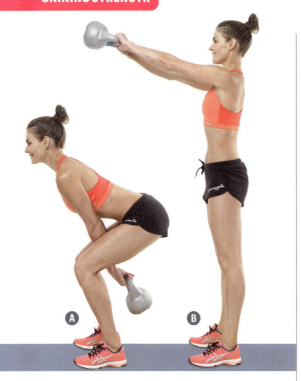

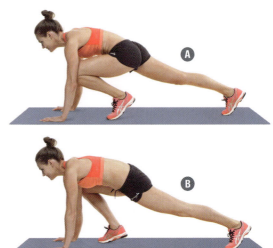

❷ MOUNTAIN CLIMBERS

▶ **Works entire body**
Get in plank position on floor with wrists aligned under shoulders and body in a straight line from head to heels. Draw left knee close to chest **[A]** then step back to start and repeat with right knee **[B]**. Once you get the feel for it, alternate driving one knee forward at a time. Try to keep body in a straight line as much as possible (don't let hips pike up). Continue for 30 seconds.

❶ KETTLEBELL SWING

▶ **Works legs, glutes, core**
Stand with feet slightly wider than shoulders and hold the handle of a 10- to 20-pound kettlebell with both hands in front of hips, palms facing body. Inhale as you bend over from the hips (back is straight) and bend your knees, swinging the kettlebell between your legs **[A]**. Quickly rise up, exhaling and powering your hips forward as you straighten your legs. Allow the momentum to drive your arms up in front of you **[B]**, no higher than your head and ideally to chest height (it may take a few reps to get the hang of it). Don't hinge forward too far or arch back when you stand up. (If you don't have a kettlebell, do this holding one end of a dumbbell in both hands.)

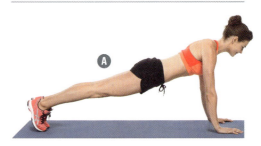

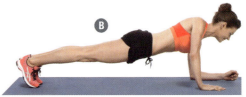

THE DEETS

▶ **WHAT TO DO** Perform 1 set of 10 to 12 reps of each move (unless otherwise noted) in order, without resting in between. After the last move, rest for 1 minute, then repeat the circuit twice.
▶ **GEAR** You'll need a pair of 8- to 10-pound dumbbells, a 10- to 20-pound kettlebell (or sub in a dumbbell), and a mat for comfort.
▶ **GET STARTED** Warm up for 5 minutes beforehand. Add cardio at the end (your choice of how long) to extend your workout time if you want.

❸ UP-AND-DOWN PLANK

▶ **Works core, triceps and shoulders**
Get in high plank position on the floor, wrists aligned under shoulders and body straight from head to heels **[A]**. (You can do this on your knees if necessary.) From high plank, lower onto left forearm **[B]** then right so both forearms are on the ground. Then press up into high plank position again, straightening left arm then right to complete 1 rep. Continue, keeping your body as straight as possible. On the next set, lead with the right arm.

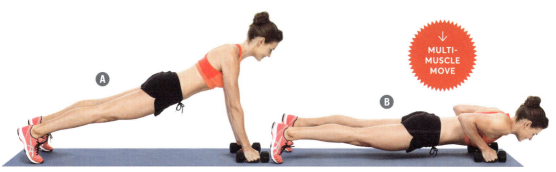

MULTI-
MUSCLE
MOVE

④ PUSH-UP TO ROW

▶ **Works chest, core, arms, back**

Hold an 8- to 10-pound dumbbell in each hand in high plank position on hands and toes, so body is straight from head to heels **[A]**. (You can do this from your knees if necessary.) Lower chest toward floor **[B]** then press up. Draw right hand toward rib cage (elbow rises above body) **[C]** then switch arms and draw left hand toward rib cage to complete 1 rep.

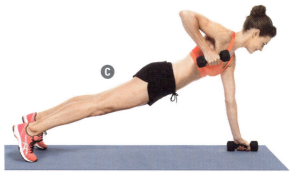

⑤ JUMPING LUNGE

▶ **Works legs, glutes and core**

Stand with feet staggered, right in front of left and lower into a lunge so right knee is aligned over right ankle **[A]** (adjust stance if necessary). Sink a little lower toward floor then jump up and switch legs **[B]**, so left leg is in front **[C]**. Jump up and switch legs again. Continue, alternating legs, for 30 seconds. Use your arms to propel you up.

CARDIO
BLAST

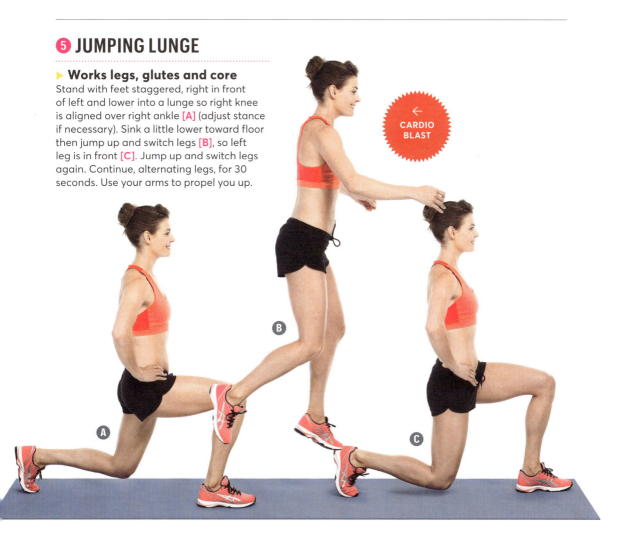

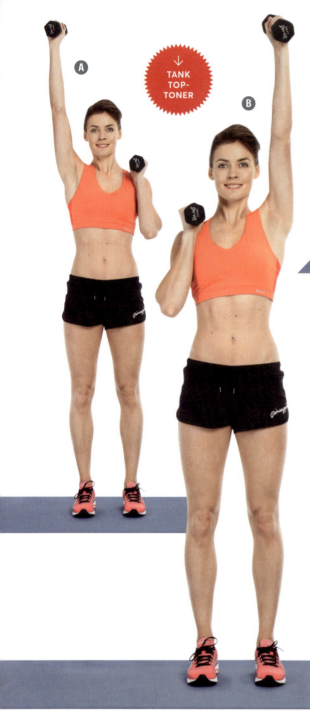

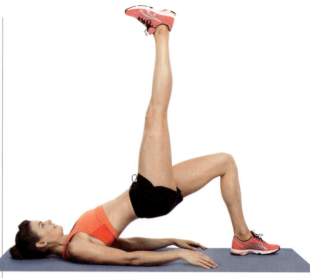

⑦ SINGLE-LEG BRIDGE

▶ **Works hamstrings and glutes**

Lie faceup with arms at sides and left leg bent, foot flat on floor. Extend right leg toward ceiling, foot flexed [shown]. Press left foot into floor as you lift hips until body is straight from shoulders to knee. Pulse leg up toward ceiling 10 to 12 times, contracting left side of glutes, then lower hips to the floor and switch sides. Keep hips squared to the floor throughout the move; don't let one side sink down or rise up.

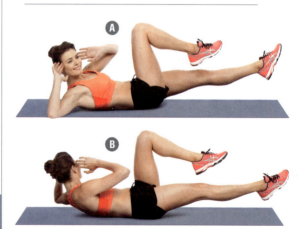

⑧ BICYCLE CRUNCH

▶ **Works abs**

Lie faceup with legs straight and hands resting lightly on either side of head (don't yank head forward). Lift head and upper back off floor, then lift legs and draw left shoulder and elbow toward right knee [A]. Switch sides, drawing right shoulder and elbow toward left knee [B]. Continue alternating sides for 1 minute. Keep legs elevated the entire time and use slow, controlled movements.

⑥ ALTERNATE SHOULDER PRESS

▶ **Works shoulders**

Stand with feet hip-width apart and hold an 8- to 10-pound dumbbell in each hand at shoulders, palms facing each other. Keeping abs engaged, press right arm up [A], then lower, and press left arm up [B] and lower to complete 1 rep. Continue, alternating sides.

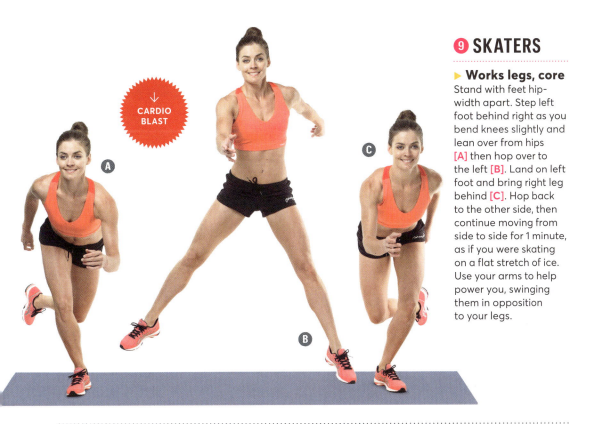

CARDIO BLAST

A

B

C

❾ SKATERS

▶ **Works legs, core**
Stand with feet hip-width apart. Step left foot behind right as you bend knees slightly and lean over from hips [A] then hop over to the left [B]. Land on left foot and bring right leg behind [C]. Hop back to the other side, then continue moving from side to side for 1 minute, as if you were skating on a flat stretch of ice. Use your arms to help power you, swinging them in opposition to your legs.

SET IT UP

Changing up your routine can be as easy as altering the tempo, rest time and number of reps and sets. These are approaches that bodybuilders sometimes use, but they can be fun to experiment with if you're a novice, too.

▶ **SLOW SETS** Just as it sounds, you take several seconds—sometimes more than 10—to lift and lower the weight. It's harder than it sounds. You may have to use a slightly lighter weight; otherwise you can get tired quickly. It's an excellent opportunity to really focus on your form but go-go-go type A's might frustrate easily using this approach.

▶ **SUPER HIGH REPS** Think 30, 60 or even 100 reps. Obviously, you need a much lighter weight for this approach. Some research has shown that you can increase muscle just as easily with this plan as with lower reps.

▶ **DROP SETS** This is a way to squeeze every last bit of oomph out of your sets and, theoretically, to target different types of muscle fibers. Instead of doing 3 sets of 12 to 15 reps, you do 1 set that way, then immediately drop the weight (say from 10-pound dumbbells to 8-pounders) and do as many reps as you can with perfect form, then immediately decrease the weight again and repeat.

Use your brain! Visualize each muscle as you are lifting.

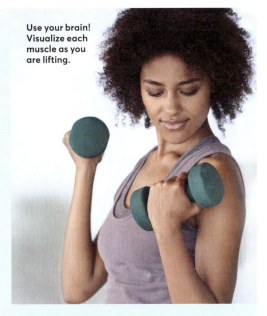

▶ **NEGATIVES** The "negative" or eccentric phase of a strength move is the part in which you're stretching the muscle under resistance—as you lower the weight during a bicep curl or the descending part of a squat. Emphasizing this phase by taking several seconds is like hitting the turbo button on your strength progress.

Pair for Super Results

Use this tactic to get leaner faster.

L et's face it: Weightlifting can be time-consuming. You do a set, then rest, then do another set, then rest. Granted, you need that recovery time for your muscles so you have full strength to go again, but you're on a tight schedule! Pairing moves back-to-back with no rest between them—called supersets—saves time without sacrificing results.

There are a few different ways to group your moves when you're supersetting: You can pair opposing muscles, like biceps and triceps; or you can pair moves that target the same muscle. A third method involves pairing upper- and lower-body moves, which can seriously rev your heart rate and metabolism.

The four supersets here primarily pair upper- (including abs) and lower-body moves. They'll have your heart pumping harder in no time. If you want to add more of a cardio kick, add a fifth superset, pairing 30 to 60 seconds of jumping jacks with 30 to 60 seconds of mountain climbers (see page 52). Soon you might be seeing double (in a good way) every time you hit the weights.

The heavier you lift, the more time you'll need to rest that muscle. For speedy workouts, use lighter weights.

Up

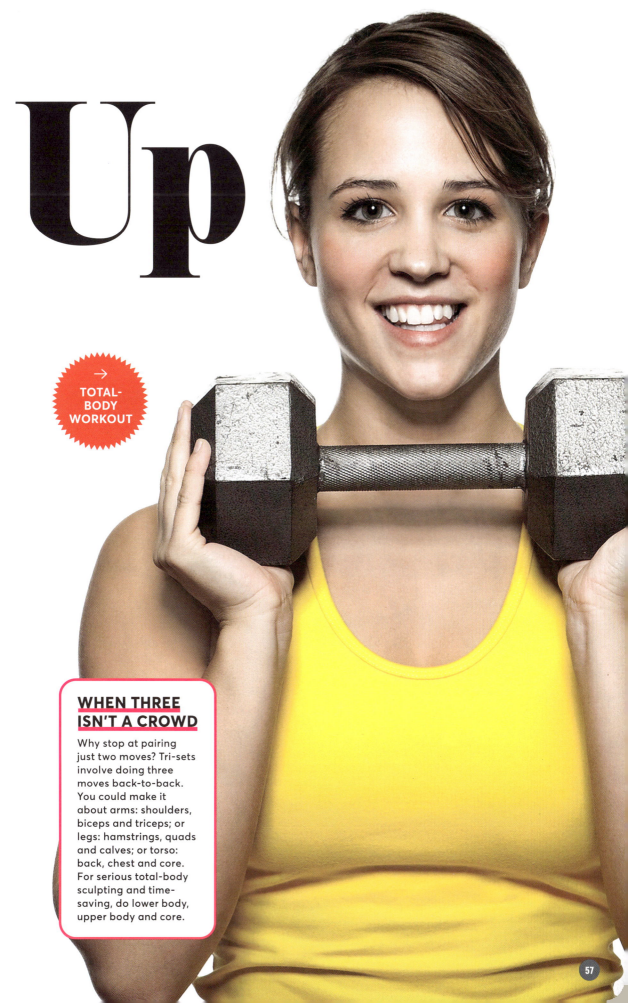

→

TOTAL-
BODY
WORKOUT

WHEN THREE ISN'T A CROWD

Why stop at pairing just two moves? Tri-sets involve doing three moves back-to-back. You could make it about arms: shoulders, biceps and triceps; or legs: hamstrings, quads and calves; or torso: back, chest and core. For serious total-body sculpting and time-saving, do lower body, upper body and core.

SUPERSET NO. 1

① SIDE LEG LIFT

▶ **Works obliques, hips and inner thighs**

Lie on your right side with legs stacked and head resting in right hand. Place left hand in front of you on floor for support [A]. Keeping your upper body still, lift legs off the floor [B], then slowly return to starting position and repeat (don't swing legs up; control the motion). Switch sides to complete set. Proceed to the next move without resting.

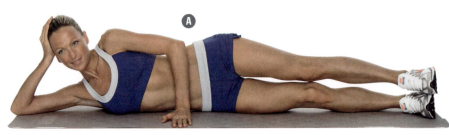

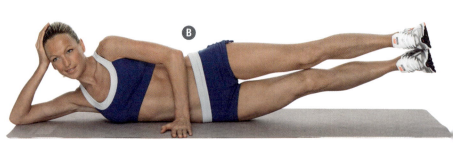

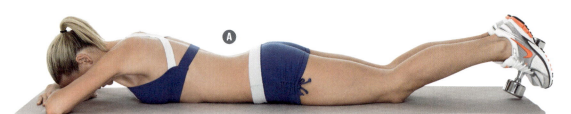

② DUMBBELL LEG CURL

▶ **Works hamstrings**

Place a 10- to 20-pound dumbbell between feet, then lie facedown (head on forearms) [A]. Squeeze your legs together then bend your knees, drawing heels toward your glutes [B]. Straighten legs to return to starting position, but keep the weight within an inch or two of the floor; repeat. Rest, then move on to Superset No. 2.

REAR-VIEW BOOSTER

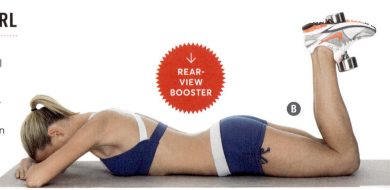

THE DEETS

▶ **WHAT TO DO** Perform 10 to 12 reps (unless otherwise noted) of each move back-to-back. Rest for a minute between supersets. Repeat series once if there's time.
▶ **GEAR** You'll need a pair of 5- to 12-pound dumbbells, one 10- to 20-pound dumbbell, and a mat for comfort.
▶ **GET STARTED** Warm up for 5 minutes beforehand.

1 SINGLE-LEG SQUAT

▶ **Works legs and glutes**

Stand with feet hip-width apart and hands on hips, then shift weight to left leg and raise right leg several inches off floor [A]. Slowly squat on left leg, as if you were going to sit in a chair behind you [B], then rise up and repeat. Switch legs to complete set. Proceed to the next move without resting.

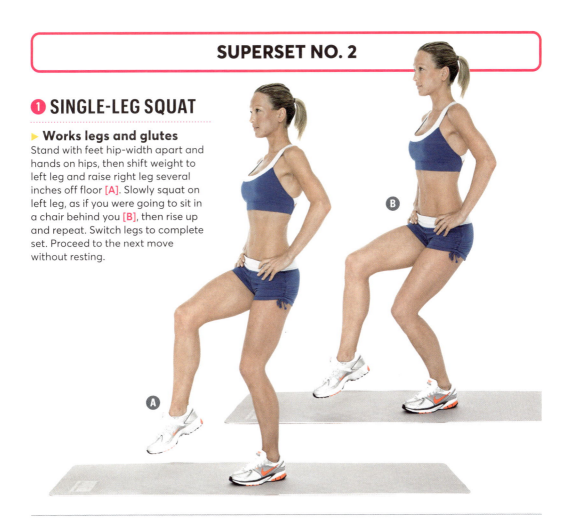

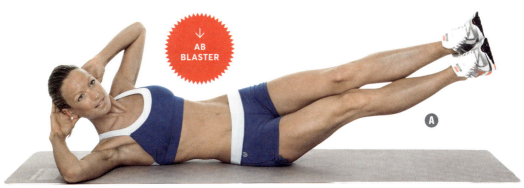

AB BLASTER

2 SIDE CRUNCH

▶ **Works abs**

Lie faceup with knees bent and hands resting gently on either side of head. Roll halfway onto right side and extend legs slightly in front of you [A]. Draw knees toward chest until left knee touches left elbow [B]. Extend legs again and repeat. Switch sides to complete set. Rest, then move on to Superset No. 3.

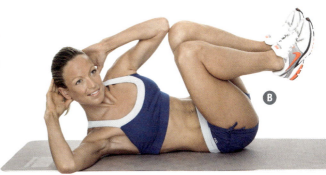

SUPERSET NO. 3

❶ PLIÉ SQUAT

▶ **Works legs, glutes and calves**
Stand with feet wider than shoulders, toes turned out, and hands on hips [A]. Keeping torso tall, bend knees out to sides and lower into a squat. Then rise up onto toes [B]. Hold for 1 count then lower heels and rise up, squeezing glutes tight; repeat. (Hold onto a chair for balance, if necessary.) To make this more challenging, hold a dumbbell in each hand. Proceed to the next move without resting.

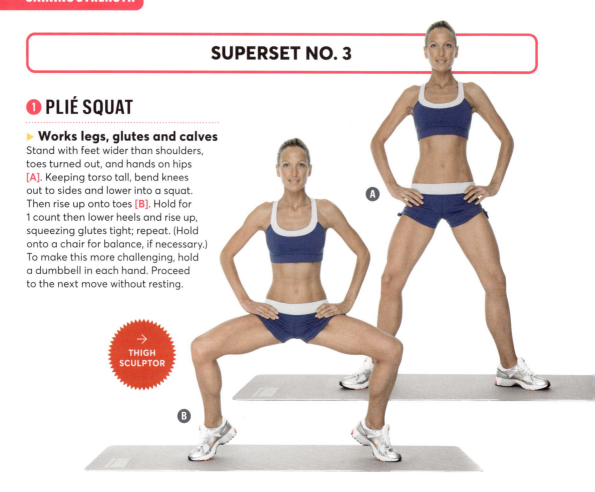

→ THIGH SCULPTOR

❷ STAGGERED PRESS-UP

▶ **Works chest, triceps and core**
Get on the floor in modified push-up position, knees down and hands under shoulders. Move right hand forward several inches and left hand back several inches so they're staggered [A]. Bend elbows and lower chest toward floor, keeping left elbow close to body while right elbow bends out to side [B]. Press up and repeat. Do 6 reps then switch arm positions and repeat. Rest, then move on to Superset No. 4.

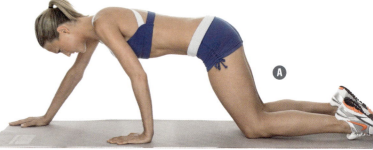

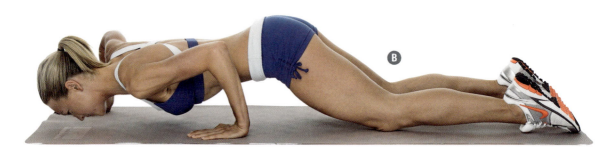

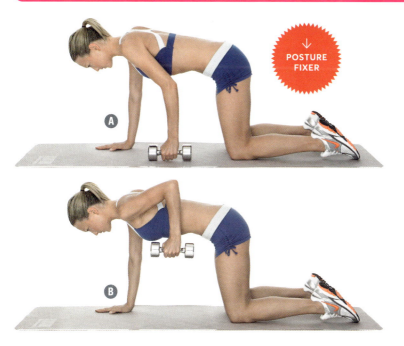

POSTURE
FIXER

❶ KNEELING ROW

▶ **Works back**

Get on all fours with a 10- to 20-pound dumbbell in left hand, aligned under left side of chest [A]. Keeping torso strong and still, bend elbow and draw weight toward chest [B]. Slowly lower to within an inch or two of the floor and repeat. Do all reps on left side, then switch arms and repeat to complete set. Proceed to the next move without resting.

❷ SQUAT TO RAISE

▶ **Works shoulders**

Stand with feet hip-width apart and hold a 5- to 12-pound dumbbell in each hand. Squat [not shown], then rise up and raise left arm parallel to floor [A]. Lower arm and raise right arm to parallel [B] to complete 1 rep. Do all reps then rest and repeat series.

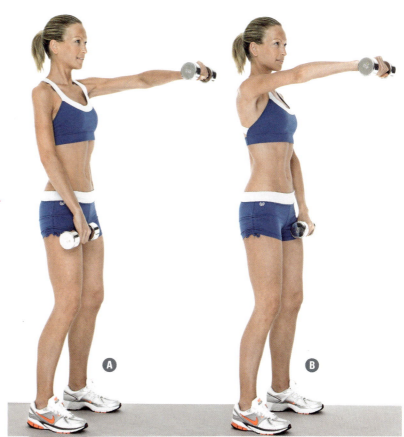

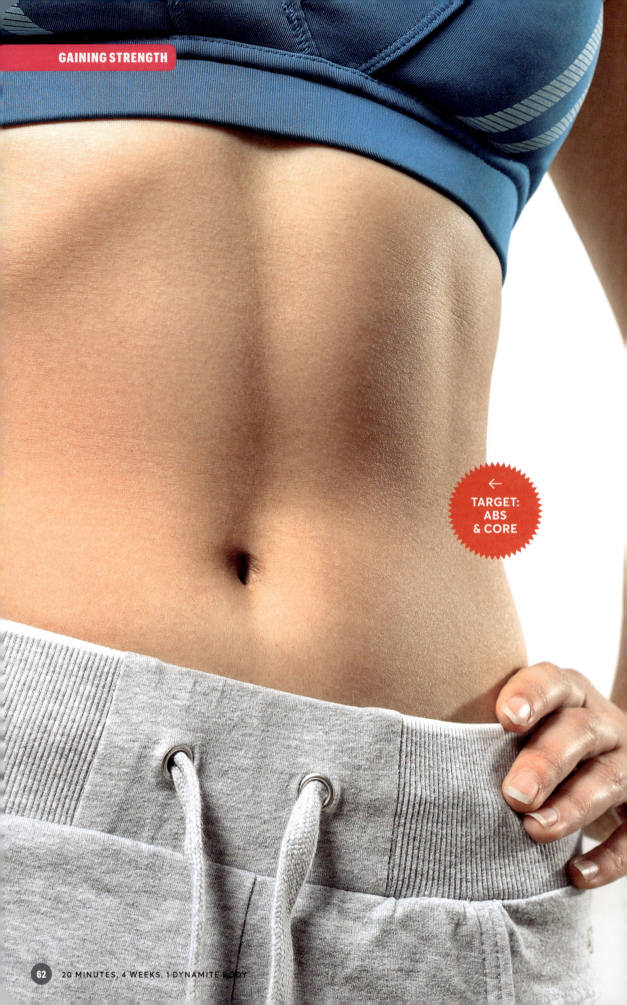

TARGET:
ABS
& CORE

Flat Abs Fast

Put a bull's-eye on your belly for a tight, toned midsection.

Paunch. Pooch. Gut. Muffin top. Spare tire. There are many different terms to refer to the extra weight you might be carrying around your midsection. And there are almost as many ways to get rid of it. Strategy No. 1: Check your diet. It's the main way to get rid of flab, no matter where it is. Next, increase your calorie burn through exercise and firm the muscles lying underneath the fat to create a stronger, firmer middle.

"I suggest using two main components: working multidimensionally (prone, supine, lateral) and adding weights or resistance," says Cindy Present, director of fitness and activities at Lake Austin Spa Resort in Texas. "That might mean using dumbbells, sandbags or resistance bands." The following workouts do just that. In addition, there are high-energy cardio blasts to spike your calorie burn as you firm. Opt for a 20-minute ab attack or use the shorter workouts when you want quick firming or an add-on to another routine. Before you know it, you'll have to find a more flattering nickname, like "six-pack," "rock" or "pancake" (as in: flat as a...).

ANATOMY LESSON

▶ **RECTUS ABDOMINIS**
This sheath runs from the bottom of the rib cage and sternum to the pubic bone.
▶ **INTERNAL OBLIQUES**
These attach at the bottom of the ribs and run back to the top of the hips.
▶ **EXTERNAL OBLIQUES**
They attach further back on the ribs and run toward the midline of the torso.
▶ **TRANSVERSE ABDOMINIS**
A deep corseting muscle, it attaches at the midline of the torso and the spine.

WORKOUT NO. 1
5-Minute Core Circuit

1 SHADOWBOXING

Stand with feet staggered, left slightly in front of right, and hold a 5- to 8-pound dumbbell in each hand on either side of jaw [A]. Punch forward with left arm then retract arm and punch forward with right, moving across the body slightly [B]. Keep your abs engaged the entire time. Continue, alternating arms, for 30 seconds, then rest for 30 seconds.

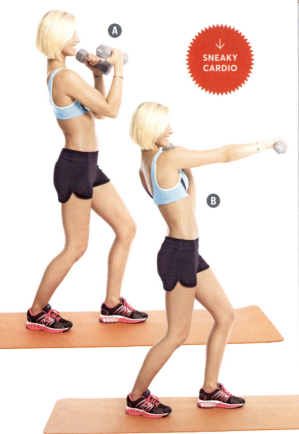

↓ SNEAKY CARDIO

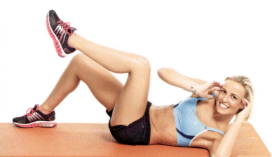

2 TWISTING CRUNCH

Lie faceup with knees bent and feet on floor, hands resting gently on either side of your head. Draw left knee in as you twist to left, bringing right elbow toward knee [shown]. Return to starting position and switch sides to complete 1 rep. Continue for 30 seconds, then rest for 30 seconds and repeat twice.

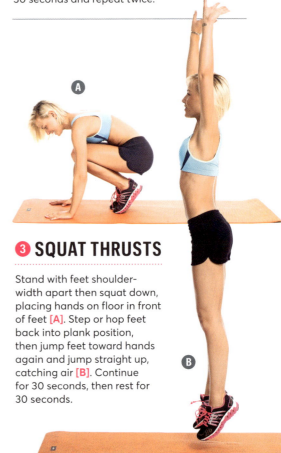

3 SQUAT THRUSTS

Stand with feet shoulder-width apart then squat down, placing hands on floor in front of feet [A]. Step or hop feet back into plank position, then jump feet toward hands again and jump straight up, catching air [B]. Continue for 30 seconds, then rest for 30 seconds.

THE DEETS

▶ **WHAT TO DO** Perform each move in order, following the time/rep instructions for each one.
▶ **GEAR** You will need a pair of 5- to 8-pound dumbbells and a mat for comfort.
▶ **GET STARTED** Warm up for 5 minutes beforehand.

WORKOUT NO. 2
10-Minute Middle Cincher

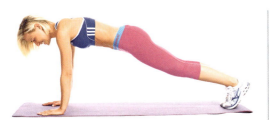

1 PLANK

Get in push-up position on hands and toes so body is straight from head to heels [shown]. Press heels behind you and press away from the mat with hands. Hold for 30 seconds, then rest for 30 seconds; repeat twice.

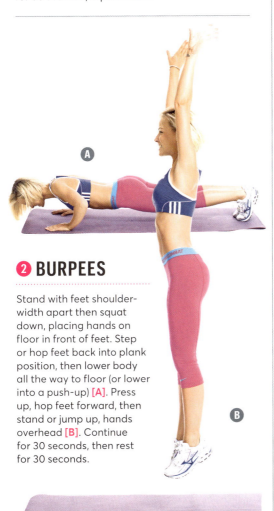

2 BURPEES

Stand with feet shoulder-width apart then squat down, placing hands on floor in front of feet. Step or hop feet back into plank position, then lower body all the way to floor (or lower into a push-up) [A]. Press up, hop feet forward, then stand or jump up, hands overhead [B]. Continue for 30 seconds, then rest for 30 seconds.

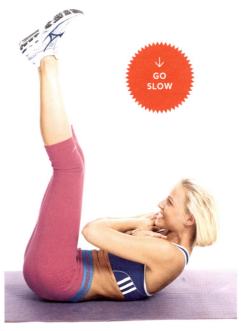

GO SLOW

3 LEGS-UP CRUNCH

Lie faceup with arms crossed over chest and legs extended over hips. Keeping legs still, lift head and upper back off floor, drawing elbows toward thighs [shown], then lower almost all the way to the floor and repeat. Use slow, controlled motion; don't jerk yourself up. Continue for 30 seconds, then rest for 30 seconds and repeat once. Repeat burpees, then proceed to No. 4.

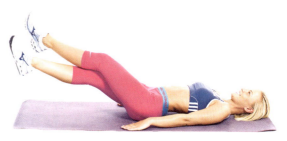

4 SCISSORS

Lie faceup with arms on floor and legs extended over hips. Draw your belly button in to keep your back from arching off the floor and slowly lower legs about 45 degrees. Keeping abs tight and head on floor, crisscross legs, one on top, then the other on top [shown], for 30 seconds. Place feet on ground and rest for 30 seconds, then repeat once. Finish with burpees.

WORKOUT NO. 3
20-Minute Belly Buster

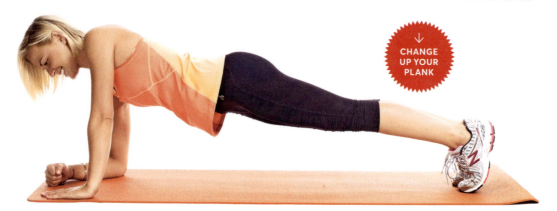

↓ CHANGE UP YOUR PLANK

1 UP-AND-DOWN PLANK

Get in plank position on hands and toes, so your body is straight from head to heels. Lower onto right forearm [shown], then left (keep elbows under shoulders), then press up onto right hand then left to complete 1 rep. On the next rep, lead with the left forearm as you lower and press up. Continue, alternating lead arms, for 30 seconds. Then rest for 60 seconds and repeat twice.

> ❝ **Target your abs from different angles and add resistance."**
> —CINDY PRESENT, LAKE AUSTIN SPA RESORT

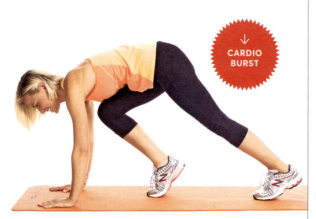

↓ CARDIO BURST

2 MOUNTAIN CLIMBERS

Get in plank position with body straight from head to heels. Draw right knee toward right arm [shown], then step back and draw left knee toward left arm. Continue, alternating legs, for 30 seconds. As you get the hang of it, jump feet back and forth and increase the speed. Rest for 30 seconds, then repeat 3 times.

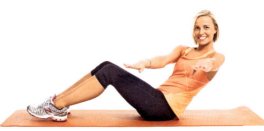

3 RUSSIAN TWIST

Sit tall on the floor with knees bent 90 degrees and feet flat. Lean back about 45 degrees and lift chest so torso is straight, not sinking toward the floor. Extend arms over knees. Twist torso to left [shown], lowering hands toward floor, then return to center and twist to right to complete 1 rep. Continue for 30 seconds, then rest for 30 seconds; repeat twice.

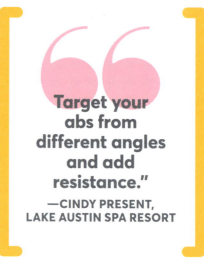

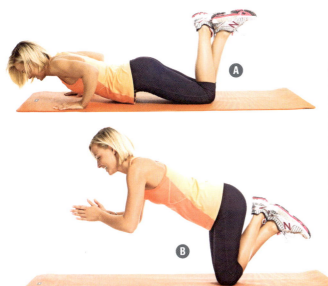

4 EXPLOSIVE PUSH-UP

Get on the floor in modified push-up position, resting on hands and knees with body straight from head to knees (bend knees and lift feet behind you with ankles crossed). Bend elbows to lower chest toward floor [A] then press up as powerfully as you can, trying to lift your hands a few inches off the floor (clap if you can [B], but you don't have to come off the floor). Slowly return to push-up and repeat. Continue for 30 seconds, then rest for 60 seconds; repeat twice.

5 REVERSE CRUNCH

Lie faceup on floor with knees bent 90 degrees and aligned over hips, arms on floor at sides [A]. Focus on the lower part of your abdominals and contract your abs to draw your knees toward your chest [B]. Slowly lower back to the start and repeat, without relying on momentum to move your legs. (If you're doing it right, you'll feel the lower part of your belly working hard!) Continue for 30 seconds, then rest for 30 seconds; repeat twice. Finish with 1 minute of mountain climbers (No. 2).

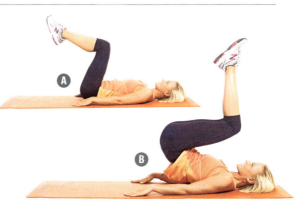

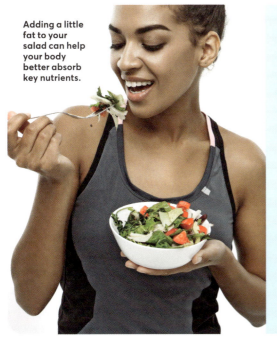

Adding a little fat to your salad can help your body better absorb key nutrients.

3 WAYS TO BURN MORE FAT

▶ **EAT RIGHT** When you're trying to cut back on calories, make sure you're not getting rid of the good stuff. Load up on healthy veggies, whole grains, lean protein and healthy fat (it still has 9 calories per gram, so be mindful). Nix the sugar, refined carbs, sodas and juices, which are sneaky sugar bombs.

▶ **BUILD MUSCLE** If you're not careful, those calories you're losing will be pulled from muscle, which you don't want. Eating adequate protein and doing strength training will help ensure that weight loss comes from fat stores.

▶ **DO HIIT** You can't "spot reduce"—or can you? Some studies have shown that when you do high-intensity interval training (HIIT), fat tends to come off the midsection first. Either way, you're burning max calories so you can't lose. Turn to page 110 for several ways to turn up your burn with HIIT.

Running and cycling are some of the best cardio exercises to help burn calories and build leg muscles.

The STEM Program

You can't control how long your legs are, but you can make them leaner and stronger.

Math and science are important topics, but the program on the next few pages is all about strengthening the stems you were born with. Your legs provide power for all your workouts, not to mention just getting around in day-to-day life. Along with your glutes (see page 72), your quadriceps and hamstrings—two primary leg muscle groups—need to be strong for things as basic as getting on and off the toilet, into and out of a car and pushing a heavy grocery cart. And if you want to get more out of your workouts, leg strength and endurance will help you go faster and longer without getting tired (your heart may feel the burn sooner than your legs will). Ready to prioritize your stem skills? The best part about this program is there are no tests to pass or formulas to remember.

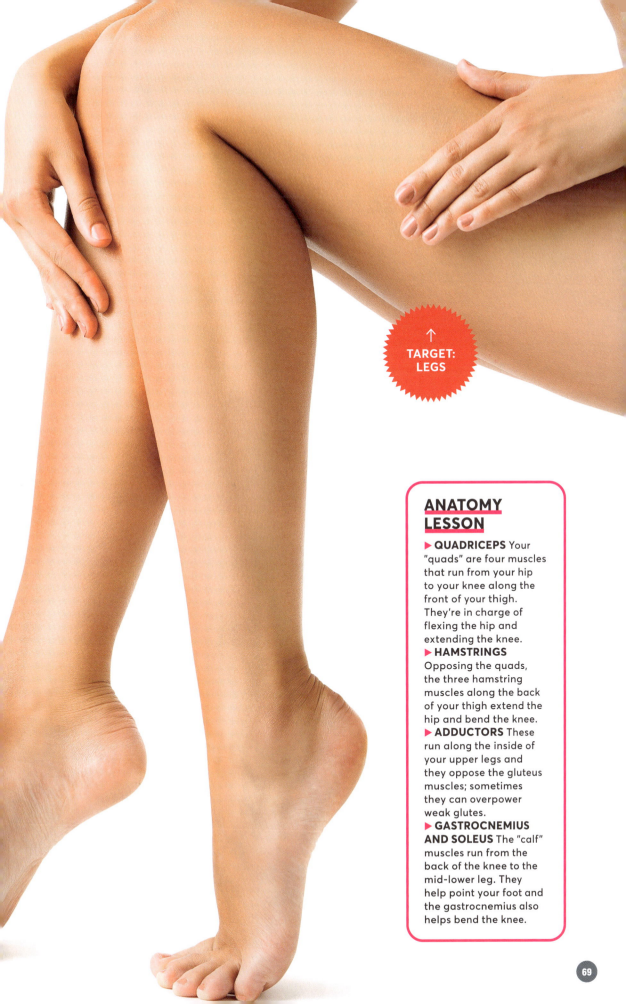

TARGET:
LESS

ANATOMY LESSON

▶ **QUADRICEPS** Your "quads" are four muscles that run from your hip to your knee along the front of your thigh. They're in charge of flexing the hip and extending the knee.

▶ **HAMSTRINGS** Opposing the quads, the three hamstring muscles along the back of your thigh extend the hip and bend the knee.

▶ **ADDUCTORS** These run along the inside of your upper legs and they oppose the gluteus muscles; sometimes they can overpower weak glutes.

▶ **GASTROCNEMIUS AND SOLEUS** The "calf" muscles run from the back of the knee to the mid-lower leg. They help point your foot and the gastrocnemius also helps bend the knee.

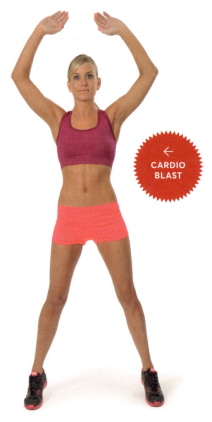

CARDIO
BLAST ←

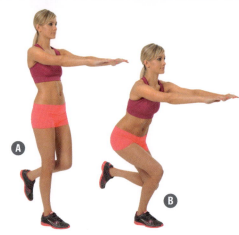

❷ SINGLE-LEG SQUAT

▶ **Works quads, glutes, hamstrings and core**
Balance on right leg with arms in front of you [A]. Slowly squat on right leg, trying to keep knee tracking over foot (don't let it angle in or out) [B]. Go as low as you can, then rise up and repeat. Do all reps on one side then switch legs to complete 1 set. Hold dumbbells at your sides for more of a challenge.

❶ JUMPING JACKS

▶ **Works quads, hamstrings, adductors, calves and shoulders**
Stand with feet hip-width apart and hands at sides. Jump feet wide as you raise arms overhead [shown], then return to starting position. Try to not let your knees track in (knock knees) as you jump wide. Make it more challenging by squatting in both positions: feet together and feet wide. Continue for 30 seconds.

❸ DUMBBELL SIDE LUNGE

▶ **Works quads, hamstrings, glutes, adductors and core**
Stand with feet hip-width apart and hold an 8- to 10-pound dumbbell in each hand in front of your thighs [A]. Lunge out to left, feet parallel, and sit back as if sitting in a chair behind you. At the same time, hinge forward from the hips and reach weights toward left foot [B]. Press off left foot to return to starting position and repeat to opposite side to complete 1 rep.

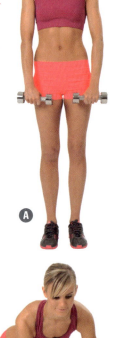

THE DEETS

▶ **WHAT TO DO** Perform 10 to 12 reps of each move in order, without resting, unless otherwise noted. After the last move, rest for 1 minute, then repeat the moves 2 or 3 times (or until 20 minutes is up). For more of a challenge, add 30 seconds of jumping jacks or jumping rope in between each exercise.
▶ **GEAR** You'll need 8- to 10-pound dumbbells and a low bench. You can do these moves without the weights or increase the weight for more of a challenge.
▶ **GET STARTED** Warm up for 5 to 10 minutes beforehand. Add cardio at the end (your choice of how long) to extend your workout time.

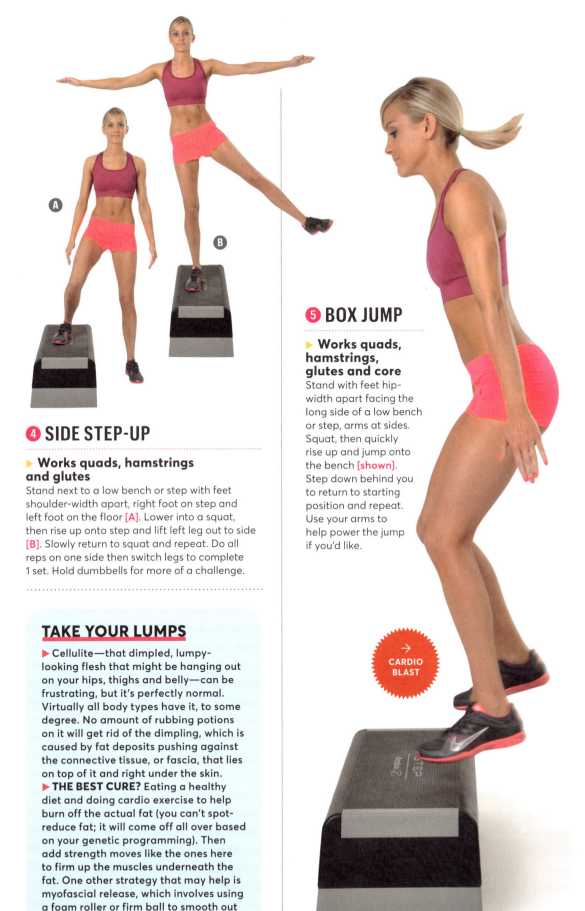

A **B**

④ SIDE STEP-UP

▶ **Works quads, hamstrings and glutes**
Stand next to a low bench or step with feet shoulder-width apart, right foot on step and left foot on the floor [A]. Lower into a squat, then rise up onto step and lift left leg out to side [B]. Slowly return to squat and repeat. Do all reps on one side then switch legs to complete 1 set. Hold dumbbells for more of a challenge.

TAKE YOUR LUMPS

▶ Cellulite—that dimpled, lumpy-looking flesh that might be hanging out on your hips, thighs and belly—can be frustrating, but it's perfectly normal. Virtually all body types have it, to some degree. No amount of rubbing potions on it will get rid of the dimpling, which is caused by fat deposits pushing against the connective tissue, or fascia, that lies on top of it and right under the skin.
▶ **THE BEST CURE?** Eating a healthy diet and doing cardio exercise to help burn off the actual fat (you can't spot-reduce fat; it will come off all over based on your genetic programming). Then add strength moves like the ones here to firm up the muscles underneath the fat. One other strategy that may help is myofascial release, which involves using a foam roller or firm ball to smooth out "kinks" or adhesions in the fascia.

⑤ BOX JUMP

▶ **Works quads, hamstrings, glutes and core**
Stand with feet hip-width apart facing the long side of a low bench or step, arms at sides. Squat, then quickly rise up and jump onto the bench [shown]. Step down behind you to return to starting position and repeat. Use your arms to help power the jump if you'd like.

→ CARDIO BLAST

Plump Your Peach

A firmer, stronger backside will help ward off back pain while making all your workouts easier.

As much as they might hate to admit it, many women *do* care about their rear view. After all, Spanx made its founder, Sara Blakely, a billionaire and household name for a reason. Some women are more self-conscious about their backside—opting for clothing that covers up their assets—while others have confidence for days. Whichever camp you're in, the important thing is that your glutes—the muscles around your hips—should be strong. (Having a firmer rear end is just a nice perk.) They help hold you upright when you're balancing on one leg (which happens with every step you take) and give you power to move. When they're weak, you run the risk of other muscles taking over, which can set you up for back and knee pain.

The moves here target your backside from a few angles, hitting the sides of the hips as well as the back, which creates a rounder, lifted look. Up the intensity by replacing rest periods with jumping jacks or jumping rope.

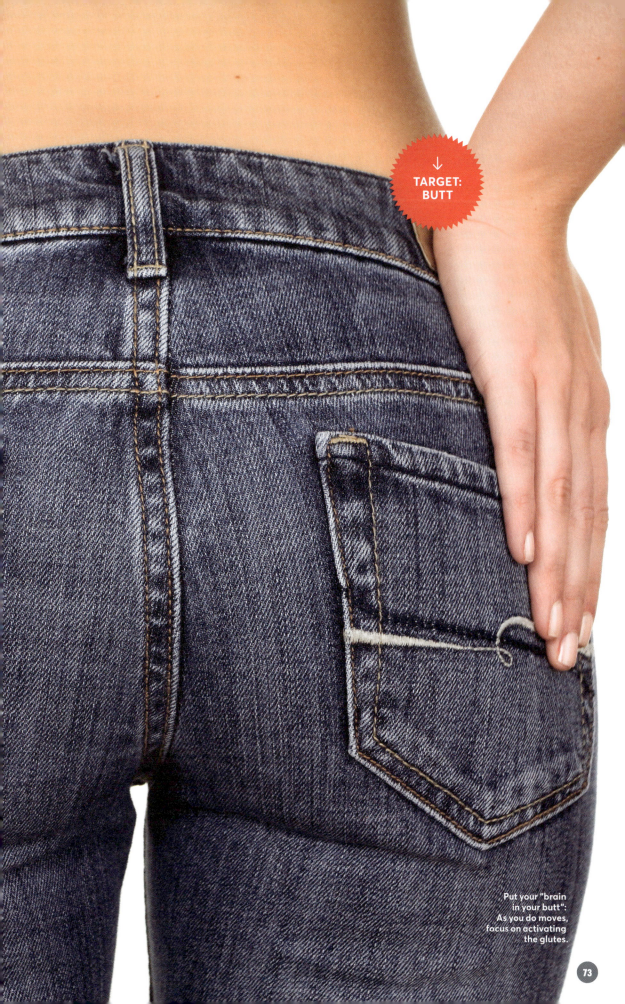

TARGET:
BUTT

Put your "brain
in your butt":
As you do moves,
focus on activating
the glutes.

THE DEETS

▶ **WHAT TO DO** Perform 3 sets of 12 to 15 reps of each move (unless otherwise noted) in order. Rest for up to a minute between sets, except with the clam and crossover kick.

▶ **GEAR** You'll need a pair of 10- to 20-pound dumbbells, a resistance band (optional) and a mat for comfort.
▶ **GET STARTED** Warm up for 5 minutes beforehand. Add

cardio at the end (your choice of how long) to extend your workout time. If you need to shorten your exercise time, you can do just 2 sets of each exercise.

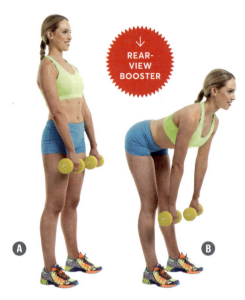

↓ REAR-VIEW BOOSTER

A   B

❶ STIFF-LEGGED DEADLIFT

Stand with feet hip-width apart and hold a 10- to 20-pound dumbbell in each hand in front of you, palms facing thighs [A]. Bend forward from the hips about 90 degrees, keeping your back straight and the weights close to your legs—almost skimming them—as you lower them toward the floor. Try to keep your knees as straight as possible [B]. Rise up to the starting position, squeezing your glutes tight as you stand up, and repeat. (For more of a challenge, do this balancing on one leg at a time.)

❷ SQUAT TO LEG RAISE

Stand with your feet hip-width apart and elbows bent at your sides (hold a dumbbell in each hand if you want an extra challenge). Toes are pointing out slightly. Squat, bending knees about 90 degrees; sit your hips back as if you were going to tap them on a stool behind you [A]. Rise up and shift your weight to your left leg as you raise your right leg and both arms out to the side [B]. Return to squat and repeat on the other side to complete 1 rep. Continue, alternating sides, until you've done 10 reps.

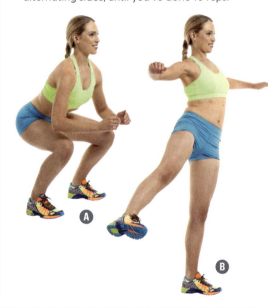

A   B

❸ CLAM

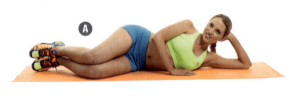

A

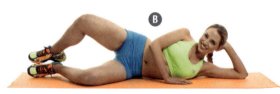

B

Lie on your left side with your back against a wall (it just keeps you from cheating). Rest your head on your left hand and bend your knees 90 degrees in front of you so just your feet and back are against the wall [A]. Keeping the inner edges of your feet together, lift your right knee away from the left as far as you can without tipping your hips back [B] (this isolates the gluteus medius). Lower the leg and repeat. Do all reps on one side, then switch and repeat to complete 1 set. For more of a challenge, place a resistance band around your lower thighs, just above the knee. You can do these sets back-to-back; rest after the last set.

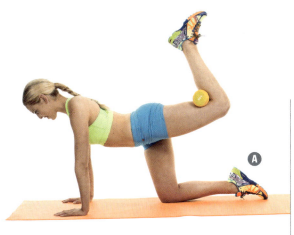

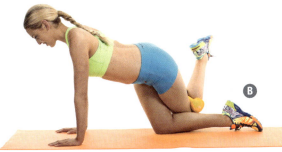

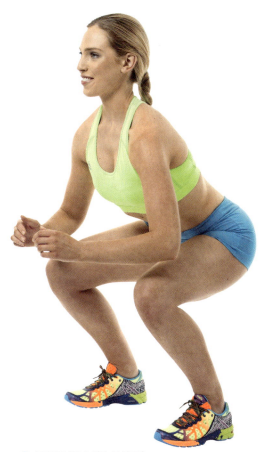

❹ CROSSOVER KICK WITH DUMBBELL

Get on all fours and tuck a 10- to 20-pound dumbbell behind your left knee. Draw your belly button in, engaging your abs, as you lift your left leg straight up, foot flexed, until thigh is parallel to the floor [A]. Lower leg to the right, crossing left knee to the outside of right leg [B]. Lift it up again and repeat. Do all reps on left side then repeat on the right to complete 1 set. You can do these sets back-to-back; rest for a minute after the last set.

❺ FINISH IT OFF!

If you have any remaining time left after you've done all your sets (no more than a minute or two), start as you did in the Squat to Leg Raise, without any dumbbells, and do squat jumps instead of raising your leg out to the side. If that's too intense, just come up onto the tip of your toes every time instead of catching air.

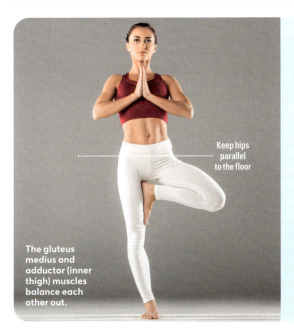

Keep hips parallel to the floor

The gluteus medius and adductor (inner thigh) muscles balance each other out.

HIP CHECK

▶ It's super common to have weak glute muscles, especially the gluteus medius. Check it with this easy test: Standing in front of a mirror, raise one leg in front of you, knee bent, to hip height (Tree Pose, like you do in yoga, will help you spot this, too). Hold here for 30 seconds as you check your hip positioning: They should be even; a yard stick placed across the top of your pelvis and resting on top of your front hip bones would be parallel to the floor.
▶ If you start to sink into your standing leg (the hip of your raised leg drops) or you notice yourself hiking up the hip on the raised leg side, your gluteus medius on the standing leg may be weak. Repeat on the other side to compare. Balancing moves and poses, like the one at left, can help strengthen these hip muscles.

Welcome to the Gun Show

Tackle your arms and upper body for results you'll want to show off all year.

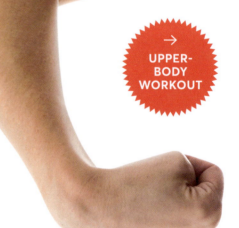

UPPER-BODY WORKOUT

Strong, defined arms (think: Michelle Obama) are the calling card of a fit body. They say, "I work out. I can carry the groceries myself. I got this." But the muscles that give those arms power—and back them up—are your chest, back and abs. These larger muscle groups are what make those push-ups or chin-ups possible. They keep your posture strong, which helps ward off aches and pains, and they help power your other workouts. It's not just about the legs, even if you're a runner or cyclist. You need upper-body strength, too.

To target all those upper-body muscles, do this workout two or three times a week. To change it up, you can add cardio intervals between each set or do the moves back-to-back in circuit format. Because it's so quick, you can pair it with lower-body moves on the same day, or alternate your days. You'll be flexing those arms in front of the mirror in no time!

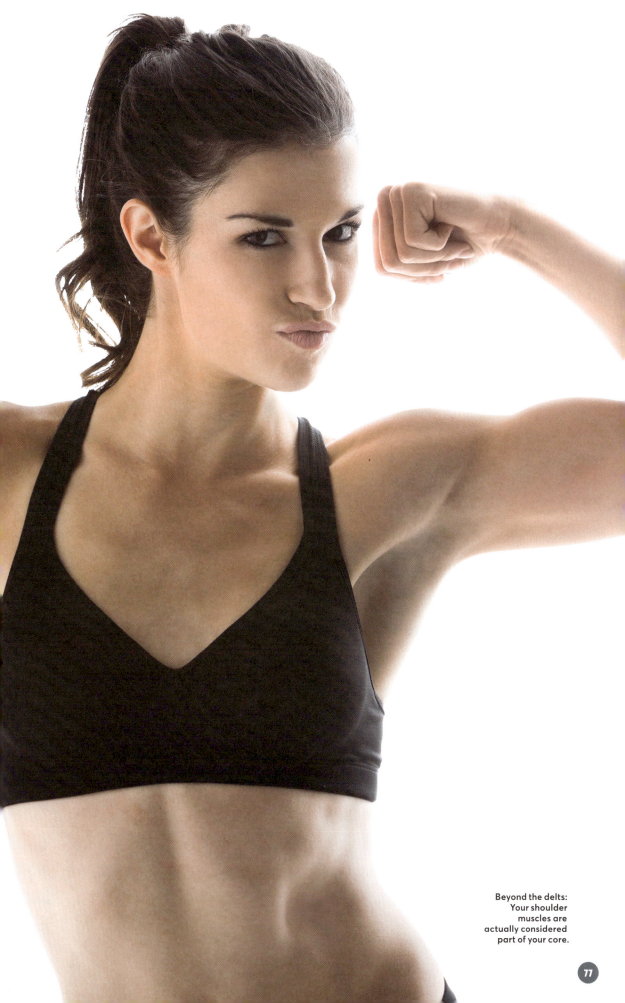

Beyond the delts:
Your shoulder
muscles are
actually considered
part of your core.

THE DEETS

▶ **WHAT TO DO**
Perform 2 sets of 10 to 12 reps of each move (unless otherwise noted), resting for up to a minute between sets (up the intensity with less rest).
▶ **GEAR** You'll need a pair of 10- to 12-pound dumbbells (you might have to go lighter for the Cuban Press) as well as a bench, sturdy chair or high step and a mat for comfort.
▶ **GET STARTED**
Warm up for 5 minutes before starting the workout.

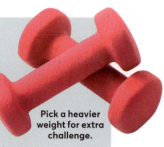

Pick a heavier weight for extra challenge.

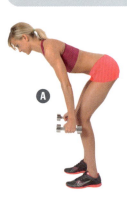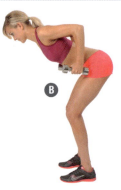

❶ DUMBBELL BENT-OVER ROW

▶ **Works back and biceps**
Stand with feet hip-width apart and hold a 10- to 12-pound dumbbell in each hand. Bend over from hips, keeping back straight, and extend arms toward floor, palms facing each other [A]. Keeping upper body still, draw weights toward sides [B]. Squeeze shoulder blades together for one count then lower and repeat.

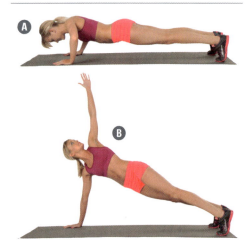

❷ T PRESS-UP

▶ **Works chest, core and triceps**
Get in high plank position on hands and toes so body is straight from head to heels. Bend elbows and lower chest toward floor [A]. Press up and lift left arm straight up, as you turn body to left [B]. Place left hand down, do a push-up, then raise right arm on next rep.

❸ DUMBBELL ZOTTMAN CURL

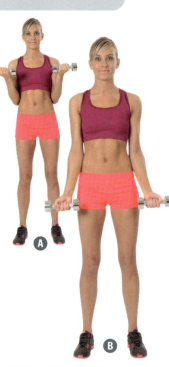

▶ **Works biceps**
Stand with feet hip-width apart and hold a 10- to 12-pound dumbbell in each hand at sides, palms facing forward. Keeping torso strong and abs engaged, bend elbows to curl weights toward shoulders [A]. Turn palms to face away from you, then lower weights toward legs to complete 1 rep. Turn palms to face forward again [B] and repeat. (To make this more challenging, squat as you curl.)

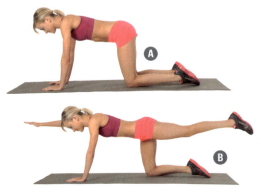

❹ QUADRUPED

▶ **Works core**
Get on all fours, wrists aligned under shoulders and knees under hips [A]. Draw belly in slightly and engage abs, then extend right arm forward and left leg back, both parallel to floor [B]. Look straight down and keep shoulders and hips squared to the floor as you hold for 1 count. Return to starting position and switch sides to complete 1 rep. Continue, alternating sides.

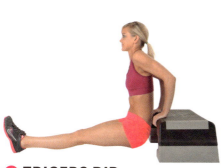

⑤ TRICEPS DIP

▶ **Works triceps, chest and shoulders**
Sit on the edge of a bench or step, palms gripping the front edge next to hips. Walk feet out until legs are straight (bend knees to make it easier), then press up and shift hips forward off bench. Keeping shoulders down, bend elbows 90 degrees, lowering hips toward floor **[shown]**. Press up and repeat.

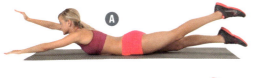

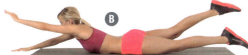

⑥ AQUAMAN

▶ **Works back and glutes**
Lie facedown with arms extended forward and legs straight. Lift head, chest, arms and legs slightly off your mat. "Swim" by lifting right arm and left leg higher **[A]**, then switch and lift left arm and right leg higher **[B]**. Continue alternating arms and legs for 30 seconds.

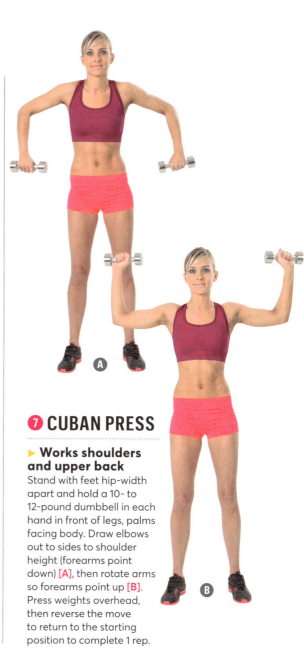

⑦ CUBAN PRESS

▶ **Works shoulders and upper back**
Stand with feet hip-width apart and hold a 10- to 12-pound dumbbell in each hand in front of legs, palms facing body. Draw elbows out to sides to shoulder height (forearms point down) **[A]**, then rotate arms so forearms point up **[B]**. Press weights overhead, then reverse the move to return to the starting position to complete 1 rep.

STOP THE SLUMP

▶ There's a name for that office slump you get: upper crossed syndrome. It's when your shoulders round forward and your chest muscles get too shortened and tight; your head comes forward; and your back muscles become overly stretched and tight. It's the perfect setup for neck and upper back pain, which are some of the most common complaints in doctors' offices.
▶ Strengthening those back muscles at the gym is key, but it can also backfire. Those large lat muscles on the sides of your back attach on the front of your upper arm bone, making them accomplices in that rounded shoulders posture. Instead, you want to make sure you're strengthening the muscles between your shoulder blades as well as the serratus anterior, which wraps around the sides of your ribs. These help keep the shoulder blades in place so you can stand up straight.

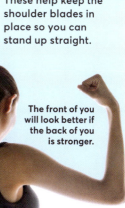

The front of you will look better if the back of you is stronger.

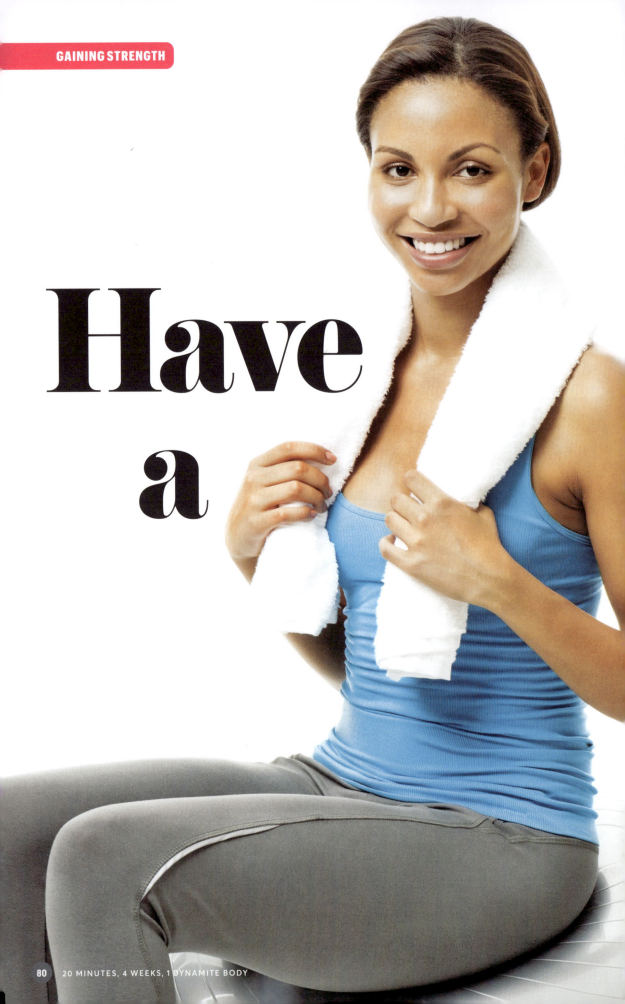

Have a

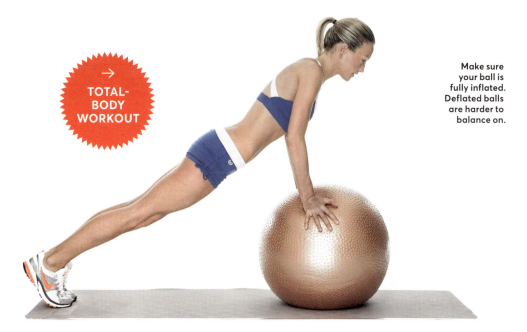

Make sure
your ball is
fully inflated.
Deflated balls
are harder to
balance on.

Ball!

Stop using it for a desk chair and incorporate it into your workout for a more well-rounded routine.

Stability balls had a moment back in the 2000s. Their sudden popularity coincided with a fascination with all things core. Doing exercises on or with the ball created anything *but* stability, forcing the muscles around your midsection to work harder. Exercise trends shift but you can still find stability balls in most gyms, and for good reason: They provide a fresh way to challenge your muscles—and you'll definitely feel it! Plus, they add a fun element to your routine—and that's always a good thing. It just feels good sometimes to splay yourself (faceup or facedown) over one of the big balls and let gravity create a nice stretch. It's like you're back in elementary school gym class.

The following moves will make your abs and back muscles work extra hard, but you'll also be targeting your chest, arms, legs and glutes. It's a total-body workout, so you can do it two or three times a week, or just sub it in for a different total-body session. Now get rolling!

PICK A SIZE

YOUR HEIGHT	BALL SIZE TO CHOOSE
Under 5'	18 inches
5'0 to 5'5"	22 inches
5'6" to 6'2"	26 inches
6'2"+	30 inches

THE DEETS

▶ **WHAT TO DO** Perform 1 set of 12 reps of each move in order, without resting. After the last move, rest for a minute, then repeat the circuit 2 or 3 more times.

▶ **GEAR** You'll need a stability ball, about 18 to 30 inches in diameter (see page 81) and a mat for comfort.

▶ **GET STARTED** Warm up for 5 minutes beforehand. Add cardio at the end (your choice of how long) to extend your workout time if you want.

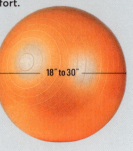

18" to 30"

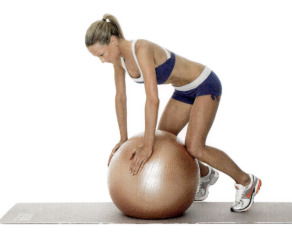

② INNER-THIGH SQUEEZE

▶ **Works inner thighs**
Stand behind ball with feet shoulder-width apart; bend knees so they're resting on sides of ball and place hands directly under shoulders on ball. (You're essentially on all-fours on the ball with feet on the ground.) Squeeze your knees toward each other, using the ball as resistance [shown]. Hold for 1 count then relax and repeat.

③ SINGLE-LEG BRIDGE

▶ **Works hamstrings, glutes and core**
Lie faceup on the floor with right knee bent and right foot resting on top of the stability ball. Extend left leg straight up and place arms at sides, palms down [A]. Press right foot into ball as you lift hips, trying to keep them square to the floor [B] (don't let one side dip down). Slowly lower your hips almost to the floor and then repeat. Do all reps on one side then switch sides to complete 1 set.

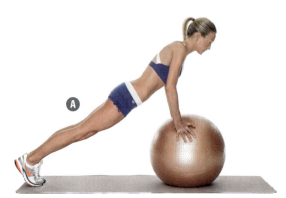

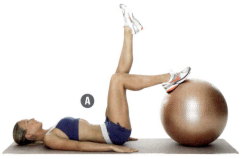

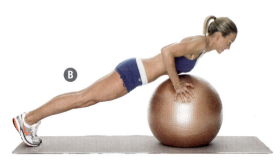

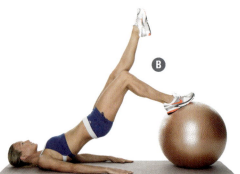

① PUSH-UP

▶ **Works chest, triceps and core**
Kneel on the floor behind a stability ball and place your hands shoulder-width apart on it. Step feet back so body is straight from head to heels and hands are aligned under shoulders [A]. Slowly bend elbows 90 degrees, lowering chest toward the ball [B], then press up and repeat. If this is too hard, lower yourself down to the ball, drop your knees to the floor then press up. (You can place the ball against a wall to make it a little easier.)

❹ COBRA

▶ Works back

Rest with your chest and abs over the ball and place your feet against a wall for balance. Extend your arms forward in a V, torso parallel to the floor [A]. Slowly bring your arms out to the sides in a T as you lift your chest off the ball [B]. Return to the starting position and repeat.

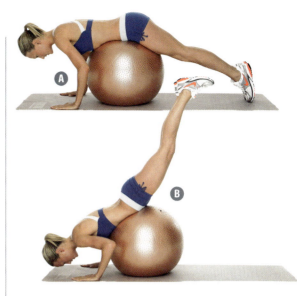

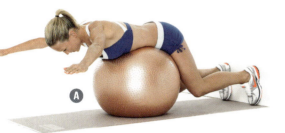

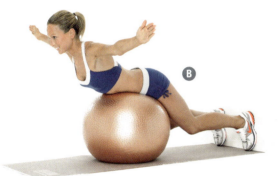

❺ REVERSE BACK EXTENSION

▶ Works lower back and glutes

Take the same starting position as in Cobra, but shift forward slightly so your arms are on the floor and legs are straight and away from the wall. Hips and lower belly should be centered on the ball [A]. Keep your upper body still as you lift your legs so they're in line with your torso [B]. (Your arms may bend more as your weight shifts forward.) Don't let your legs lift so far that your back arches. Slowly lower your legs to the floor and repeat.

❻ OBLIQUE CRUNCH

▶ Works obliques

Position your body perpendicular to the ball with your right side on it (your belly button should be directly over the center); stagger your feet against a wall or staircase for balance. Place hands behind head or in front of chest [A]. Keeping legs still, lift upper body away from ball [B], then lower and repeat. Do all reps on one side then switch sides to complete 1 set. Rest before going back to move No. 1.

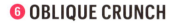

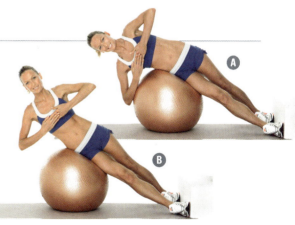

"ORB" IT

Add these three other balls to your routine for a strengthening boost.

▶ **MEDICINE BALL** These come in a variety of weights and sizes, hard rubber or padded. You can use them for weighted crunches, tossing them against a wall, Russian twists, pullovers, partner tosses and more.

▶ **SLAM BALL** Still weighted (often with sand), these are mushier, making them ideal for throwing on the floor because they won't bounce back and smack you in the face like other types of medicine balls will. Instead, you have to squat down and pick them up each time.

▶ **PILATES BALL** Filled with air and in different sizes, these add an extra challenge to Pilates moves. You can lay back over them, squeeze them between your legs or use them in a variety of other ways.

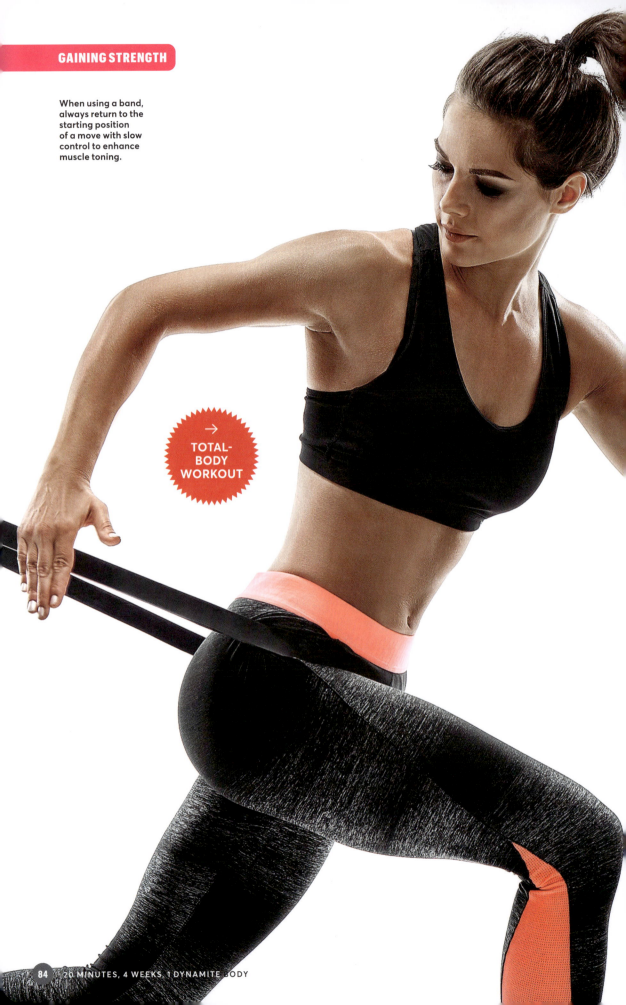

When using a band, always return to the starting position of a move with slow control to enhance muscle toning.

→ TOTAL-BODY WORKOUT

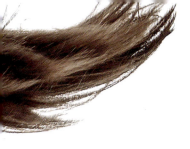

Get With the Band

Stretchy resistance is super convenient and provides a new challenge for muscles.

Resistance bands are the ultimate workout excuse-buster. No space to store weights? Travel all the time? Stuck at work all day? No problem! All you need is a resistance band, which tucks easily into a drawer, tote bag or suitcase. Bands allow you to work with resistance in the same way weights do, but with one key difference: The tauter the band gets (the more elongated it is), the more challenging it becomes. You can do many of the same moves as you would with weights—and more. Since you can anchor it on things (make sure it's secure), you can be more creative with moves as well.

If you're a newbie to using bands, these moves will help you get the feel for how they work. One thing to keep in mind: Keep a tight grip on the ends and make sure you're using a band that hasn't been stuffed in a drawer for years. As rubber ages, it gets little tears and is more likely to rip as you're using it. Oh, snap!

THE DEETS

▶ **WHAT TO DO** Perform 1 set of 12 reps of each move in order, without stopping, then finish with a minute of jumping jacks. Rest for up to a minute, then repeat the circuit 3 more times.
▶ **GEAR** You'll need a flat resistance band and a mat for comfort. Tension varies by color and also by company. Yellow, orange and red are often on the easier end; darker colors, like black or dark blue, are usually more challenging.
▶ **GET STARTED** Warm up for 5 minutes beforehand. Add cardio at the end (your choice of how long) to extend your workout time if you want.

❶ SQUAT WITH BAND

▶ **Works legs and glutes**
[not shown] Stand with feet shoulder-width apart on the center of the resistance band. Hold an end in each hand next to shoulders, elbows bent and palms facing forward. The band should be taut here; if it's not, choke up on the band more by wrapping it around your hands again. Squat, shifting your hips back as if sitting in a chair behind you. Rise up, squeezing your glutes tight as you do, and repeat. For more of a challenge—and if the band is long enough—extend arms overhead as you rise up.

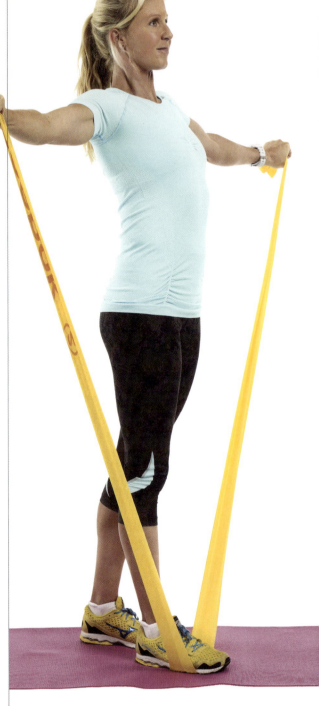

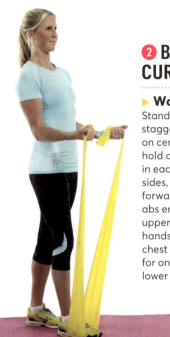

❷ BICEPS CURL

▶ **Works biceps**
Stand with feet slightly staggered, front foot on center of band and hold an end of the band in each hand at your sides, palms facing forward. Keeping your abs engaged and upper arms still, curl hands toward your chest [shown]. Hold for one count, then lower and repeat.

❸ STANDING LATERAL RAISE

▶ **Works shoulders**
Stand with feet slightly staggered, front foot on center of band, and hold an end of the band in each hand at your sides, palms facing thighs. Keeping your shoulders down, elbows slightly bent and abs tight, raise arms out to sides to shoulder height [shown]. Hold for 1 count, then lower arms and repeat.

❹ SEATED ROW

▶ Works back and biceps

Sit with center of band wrapped around arches of feet so it won't pop out. Hold an end of band in each hand, palms facing each other, and extend arms toward feet. Band should have no slack at this point. Sit tall and draw elbows behind you, squeezing shoulder blades together and lifting chest [shown]. Hold for one count, then slowly release and repeat.

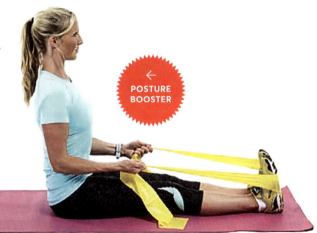

← POSTURE BOOSTER

❺ TRICEPS EXTENSION

▶ Works triceps

Stand with right foot on one end of band and hold the other end in right hand. Raise right arm overhead and bend elbow so hand rests behind head and elbow points up. Band should be straight but not taut here. Keeping upper arm still and abs engaged, straighten arm overhead [shown]. Hold for 1 count then lower and repeat. Do all reps, then switch arms to complete set. Finish with a minute of jumping jacks.

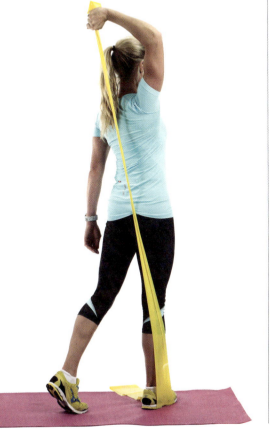

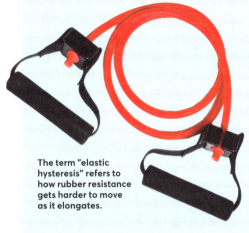

The term "elastic hysteresis" refers to how rubber resistance gets harder to move as it elongates.

PICK YOUR STYLE

Rubber resistance comes in a variety of styles that can be fun to experiment with. Try on the following for size.

▶ **HANDLED RESISTANCE TUBES** The handles make these easier to hold on to, but otherwise they work just like resistance bands. Instead of choking up on the tubing, you can loop it around your anchor point or step back to increase the resistance.

▶ **MINI BANDS** Back in the day, you had to tie a knot in the flat resistance band to make a loop. Now they come in circles, which make them great for upper- and lower-body resistance work. Just loop them around your lower arms, upper legs, shins or ankles.

▶ **FABRIC RESISTANCE BANDS** Worried about the tube getting damaged or snapping? Brands like FitCords encase the band in stretchy fabric. That way if they pop, they won't smack you in the face.

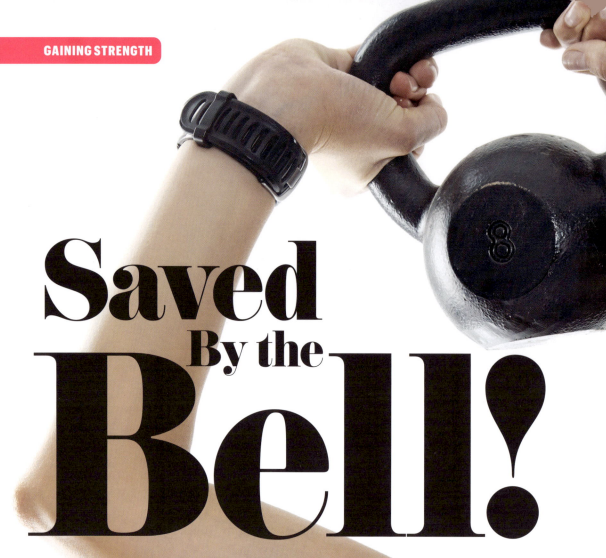

Saved By the Bell!

The versatility of this cannonball-like contraption may just turn you into a "swinger."

They may come in fun hues like pink, blue and green, but don't be fooled: Kettlebells are made for hard-core strength work. Sure, you can use them just like you would use a dumbbell for standard exercises like curls or weighted crunches, but the design allows you to use them for more powerful moves (see the Swing, page 90) as well. Those kinds of exercises drive up your heart rate and make your muscles work harder, so you get a more intense workout. (That makes them a fun addition to a weight circuit when you're trying to keep your heart rate up.) In addition, when you hold onto the handle, the heaviest part of the kettlebell can still move around, forcing you to engage more muscles to try to control it. That doesn't happen when you hold a dumbbell. Finally, when you're working with kettlebells, you're often using a weight that's heavier than you're used to, so form is key to protect yourself (see "Fix Your Form," far right). Now grab a 'bell and get swinging!

Padded wrist bands can protect your arms from the weight during certain exercises.

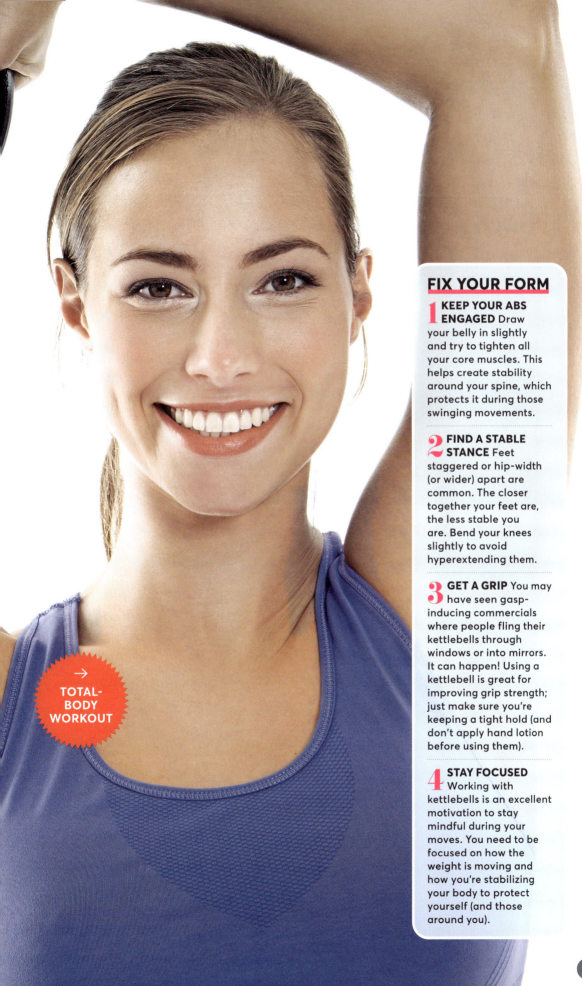

TOTAL-BODY WORKOUT

FIX YOUR FORM

1 KEEP YOUR ABS ENGAGED Draw your belly in slightly and try to tighten all your core muscles. This helps create stability around your spine, which protects it during those swinging movements.

2 FIND A STABLE STANCE Feet staggered or hip-width (or wider) apart are common. The closer together your feet are, the less stable you are. Bend your knees slightly to avoid hyperextending them.

3 GET A GRIP You may have seen gasp-inducing commercials where people fling their kettlebells through windows or into mirrors. It can happen! Using a kettlebell is great for improving grip strength; just make sure you're keeping a tight hold (and don't apply hand lotion before using them).

4 STAY FOCUSED Working with kettlebells is an excellent motivation to stay mindful during your moves. You need to be focused on how the weight is moving and how you're stabilizing your body to protect yourself (and those around you).

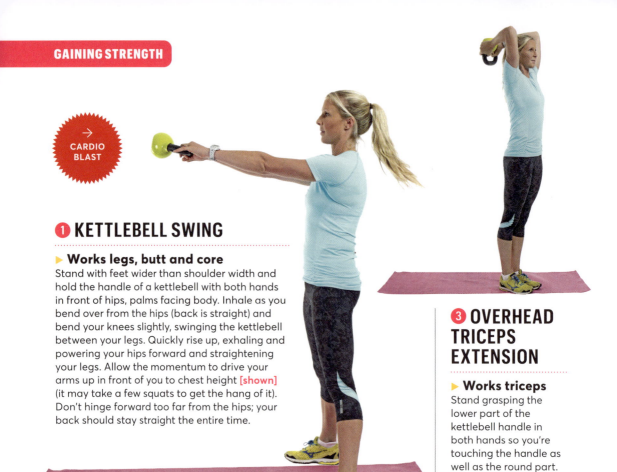

CARDIO BLAST →

❶ KETTLEBELL SWING

▶ **Works legs, butt and core**

Stand with feet wider than shoulder width and hold the handle of a kettlebell with both hands in front of hips, palms facing body. Inhale as you bend over from the hips (back is straight) and bend your knees slightly, swinging the kettlebell between your legs. Quickly rise up, exhaling and powering your hips forward and straightening your legs. Allow the momentum to drive your arms up in front of you to chest height [shown] (it may take a few squats to get the hang of it). Don't hinge forward too far from the hips; your back should stay straight the entire time.

❸ OVERHEAD TRICEPS EXTENSION

▶ **Works triceps**

Stand grasping the lower part of the kettlebell handle in both hands so you're touching the handle as well as the round part. Extend arms overhead, then, keeping upper arms close to your ears and abs engaged, bend elbows and slowly lower weight behind head [shown]. Raise arms overhead again and repeat.

❷ RENEGADE ROW

▶ **Works core and back**

Get in high plank position on the floor—wrists under shoulders and legs straight—with the kettlebell next to your right hand. Grab the kettlebell handle with right hand and draw it toward rib cage (elbow rises behind you) [shown]. Lower it and repeat. Do 8 to 10 reps on one side, then switch arms to complete set. Keep your hips and shoulders squared to the floor as much as possible. Lower to your knees if you need to.

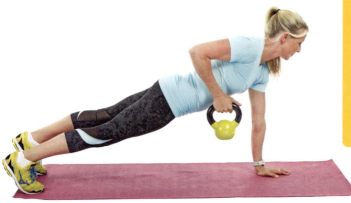

20

Calories you can burn a minute doing a kettlebell workout, per research by the American Council on Exercise

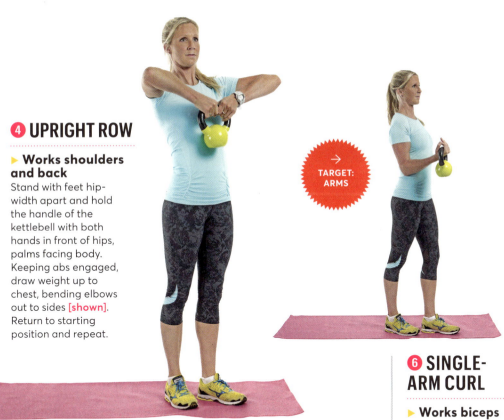

4 UPRIGHT ROW

▶ **Works shoulders and back**

Stand with feet hip-width apart and hold the handle of the kettlebell with both hands in front of hips, palms facing body. Keeping abs engaged, draw weight up to chest, bending elbows out to sides [shown]. Return to starting position and repeat.

TARGET: ARMS

5 ONE-ARM CHEST PRESS

▶ **Works chest**

Lie faceup on the floor with knees bent and feet flat, and hold the kettlebell handle with right palm facing away from you and arm extended straight over chest [shown]. Bend elbow out to side and lower kettlebell next to chest, then press it straight up again. Do all reps with right arm then switch sides to complete set.

6 SINGLE-ARM CURL

▶ **Works biceps**

Stand with feet hip-width apart or staggered and hold the kettlebell handle in right hand at your side, palm facing forward. Keeping upper arm still, curl weight toward your shoulder [shown]. Slowly lower to starting position and repeat. Do all reps on one side then switch arms (and foot position if feet are staggered) to complete 1 set.

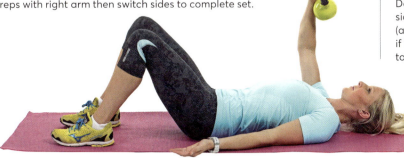

THE DEETS

▶ **WHAT TO DO**
Perform 1 set of 12 reps of each move in order, without resting. After the last move, rest for a minute, then repeat the circuit up to three times. (If you need a break earlier, take it.)

▶ **GEAR** You'll need a mat and a 10- to 15-pound (4 to 7 kg) kettlebell; you may want a heavier one for the Swing, Renegade Row and Upright Row. You can sub in a dumbbell for any of

these. For the swing, just hold the dumbbell around one end.
▶ **GET STARTED**
Warm up for 5 minutes beforehand. Add cardio at the end to extend your workout time, if you'd like.

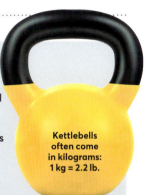

Kettlebells often come in kilograms: 1 kg = 2.2 lb.

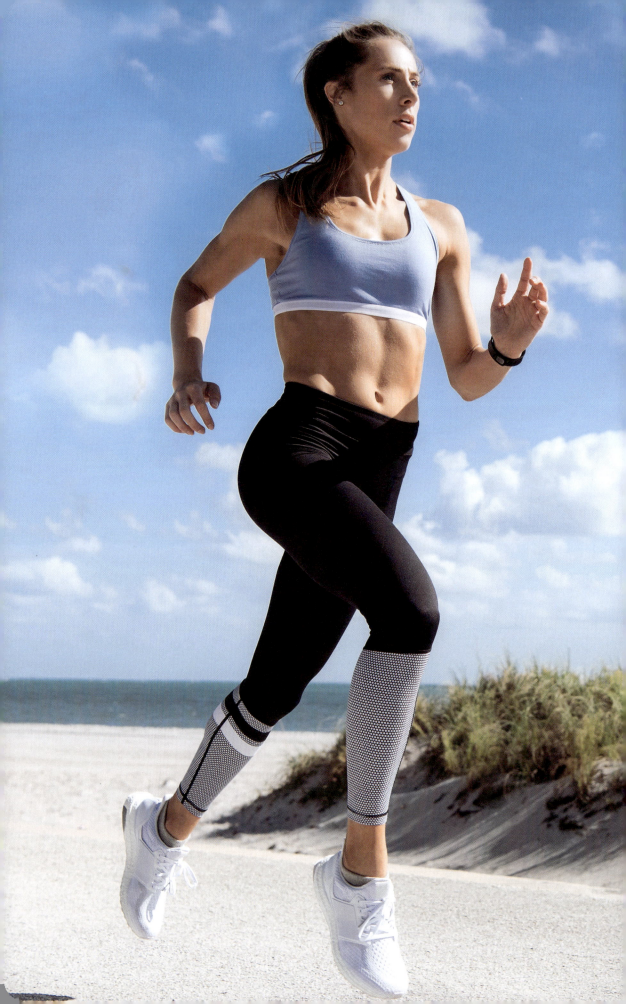

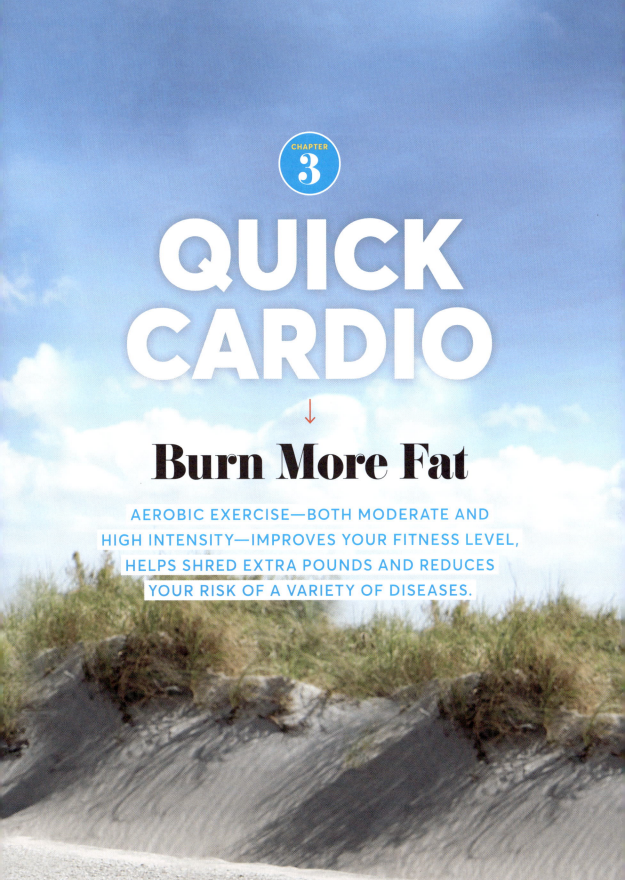

CHAPTER **3**

QUICK CARDIO

↓

Burn More Fat

AEROBIC EXERCISE—BOTH MODERATE AND
HIGH INTENSITY—IMPROVES YOUR FITNESS LEVEL,
HELPS SHRED EXTRA POUNDS AND REDUCES
YOUR RISK OF A VARIETY OF DISEASES.

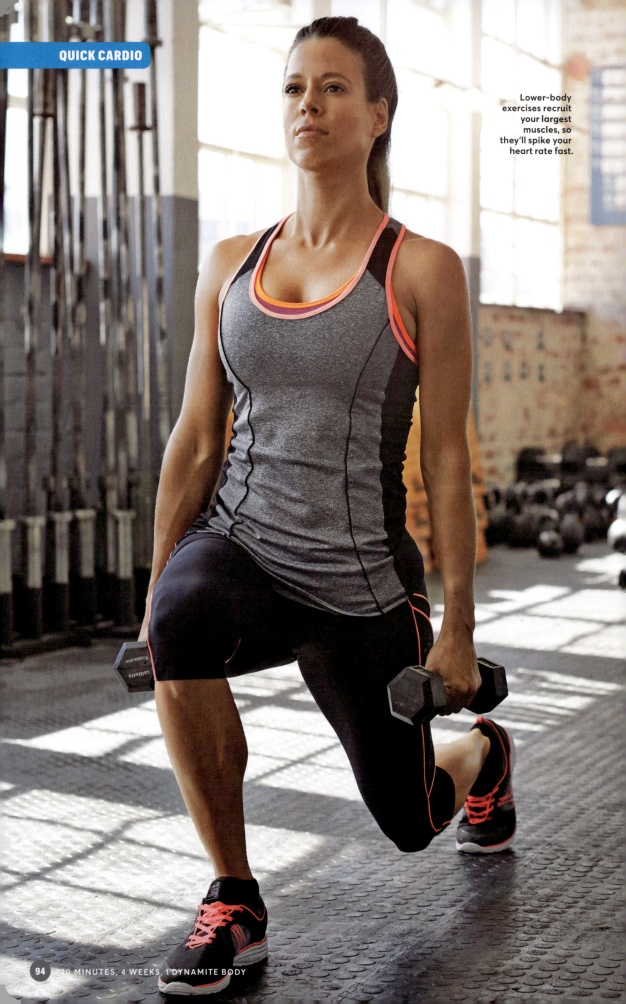

Lower-body exercises recruit your largest muscles, so they'll spike your heart rate fast.

Circuit City

Having exercise ADD can work in your favor, helping you burn more calories and speed up a boring routine.

Moving quickly from exercise to exercise—whether it's cardio, strength or a combo of both—is called circuit training. It cuts out (or shortens) rest periods and turns up the intensity of any workout. If you've flipped through the many routines in Chapter 2, you may have noticed that virtually all of those programs can be done in circuit fashion. You can do the moves back-to-back (only resting after the last exercise) or you can substitute those rest breaks with brief, higher-intensity cardio exercises. Either way, combining strength with cardio is the ultimate time-saving workout, says L.A.–based fitness and wellness coach Patricia Friberg. "You're not shortchanging either one," she says. "If you only have 20 minutes, it's a great way to boost your metabolism and calorie burn."

One caveat: If you're lifting heavy weights with an eye toward building muscle, you'll need adequate rest time to recover after each set, so circuits are best done on those days when you're not using a ton of weight. But if your calendar (and workouts) could use some streamlining, try one of these speedy twofer sessions, which will take you through a complete routine in a flash.

THE DEETS

▶ **WHAT TO DO** Choose one of the following four workouts, 2 to 3 times a week.
▶ **GEAR** You'll need a pair of 5- to 12-pound dumbbells and a jump rope for some of these.

WORKOUT NO. 1
Outdoor Circuit

Dying to get some fresh air while you exercise? Head to your backyard or nearest park for this plan. Bring a jump rope (if you have one) and use it as an option for your cardio bursts. You can take this routine indoors to a cardio machine as well, including the rower or group-cycling bike. (Use a machine that you can just jump on and go, not one that needs programming or takes time to get up to full speed.) Keep your intensity at moderate to somewhat hard throughout this program (versus the high-low approach in HIIT).

MINUTES	WHAT TO DO
0–5	Warm up with a fast walk or easy jog
5–6	Walking lunges
6–7	Walk/jog/jump rope
7–8	Push-ups on a bench or playground equipment
8–9	Walk/jog/jump rope
9–10	Squats
10–11	Walk/jog/jump rope
11–12	Crunches
12–13	Walk/jog/jump rope
13–14	Burpees
14–15	Walk/jog/jump rope
15–16	Step-ups on a bench or step
16–17	Walk/jog/jump rope
17–18	Hold plank (rest briefly if necessary)
18–20	Walk it out to cool down

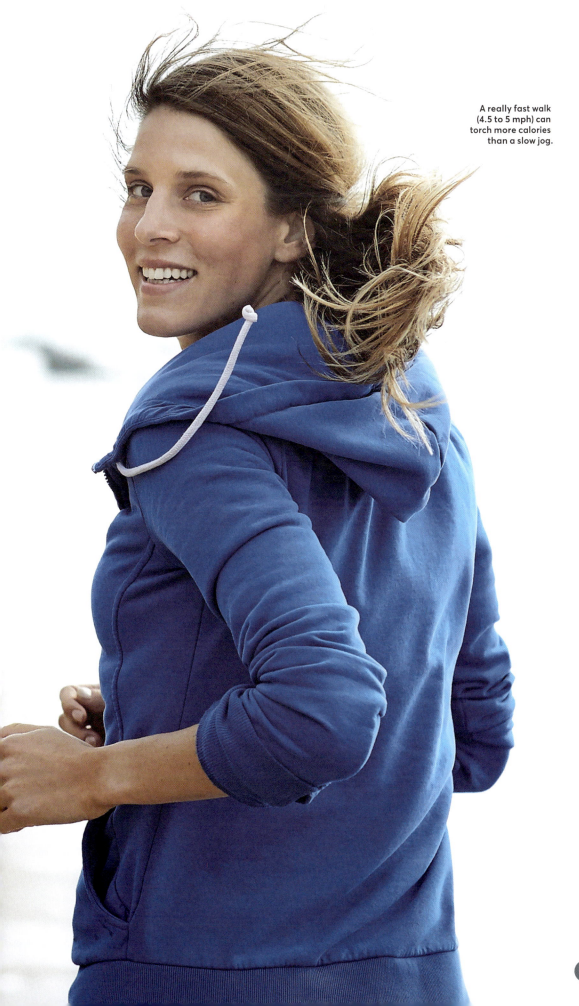

A really fast walk
(4.5 to 5 mph) can
torch more calories
than a slow jog.

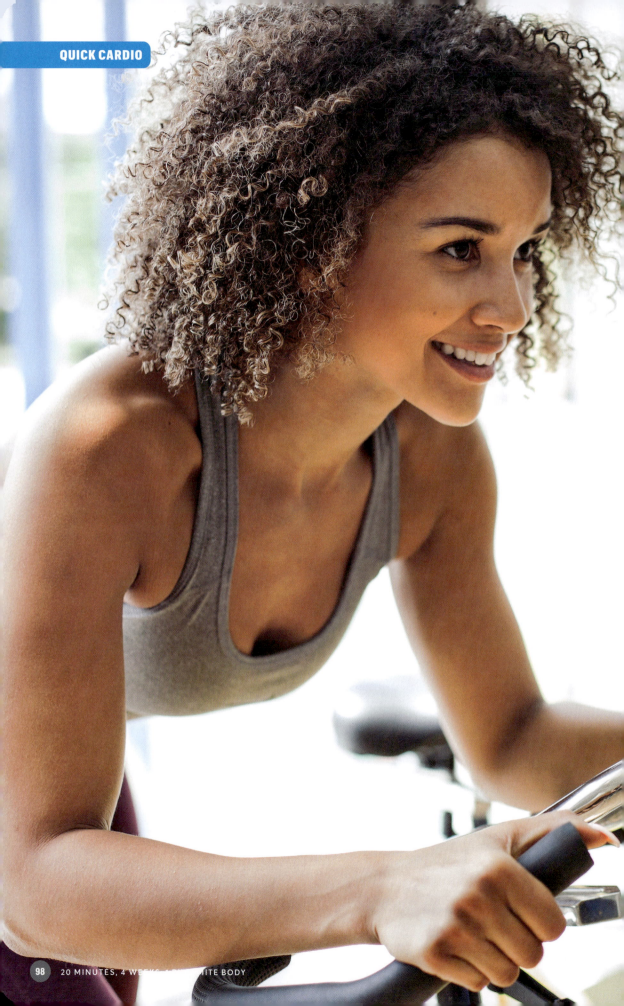

WORKOUT NO. 2
Machine Circuit

This session takes advantage of those cardio machines at the gym, with an eye toward busting boredom. DIY at home if you have a bike, jump rope or a cardio machine. Adjust the incline/resistance to maintain the noted intensity (see box at right).

MINUTES	WHAT TO DO	INTENSITY/RPE
0–3	Treadmill: Warm up with a fast walk	Easy to moderate/2–4
3–8	Jump on the bike, alternating flats (in the saddle) and climbs every 30 seconds, maintaining the same intensity	Moderate to somewhat hard/5–7
8–13	Switch to the rowing machine. See if you can hit 1,000 meters in these 5 minutes	Somewhat hard/6–7
13–18	Jump on the stair machine or elliptical	Moderate to somewhat hard/6–7
18–20	Take it back to the treadmill and finish with an easy jog	Easy/2

CHECK YOURSELF

Gauge your effort using this rating of perceived exertion (RPE) scale.

INTENSITY	RPE
Very Light	0-1
Light	2
Moderate	3-6
High	7-8
Very High	9
Maximum	10

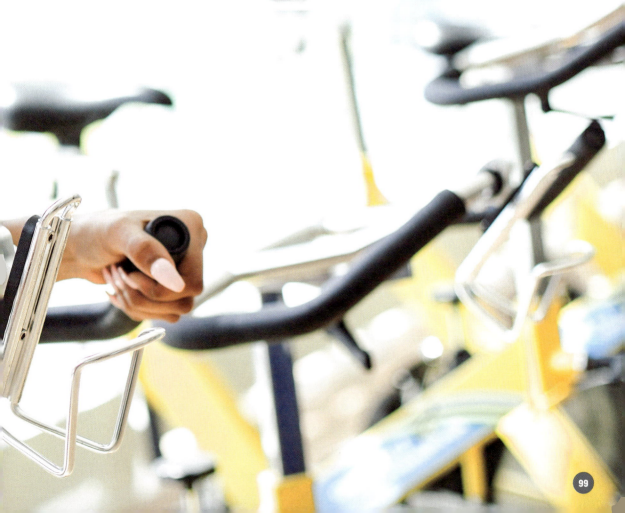

WORKOUT NO. 3
Strength Circuit

Use the moves from the Gaining Strength section of this book (page numbers are noted) for this workout. You'll do three moves in a row followed by a minute of cardio. Your intensity should stay pegged at moderate to somewhat hard during this entire workout.

MINUTES	WHAT TO DO	PAGE NUMBER
0–5	Warm up with a fast walk or easy jog	
5–6	Stiff-legged deadlift	p. 74
6–7	Clam	p. 74
7–8	Box jump	p. 71
8–9	Jump rope or jog in place	
9–10	Up-and-down plank	p. 66
10–11	Russian twist	p. 66
11–12	Reverse crunch	p. 67
12–13	Jump rope or jog in place	
13–14	Push-up to row	p. 53
14–15	Alternate shoulder press	p. 54
15–16	Triceps dip	p. 79
16–17	Jump rope or jog in place	
17–18	Plyo lunge	p. 119
18–20	Walk it out to cool down	

Jumping rope burns about 10 calories a minute. Up the tally with faster footwork.

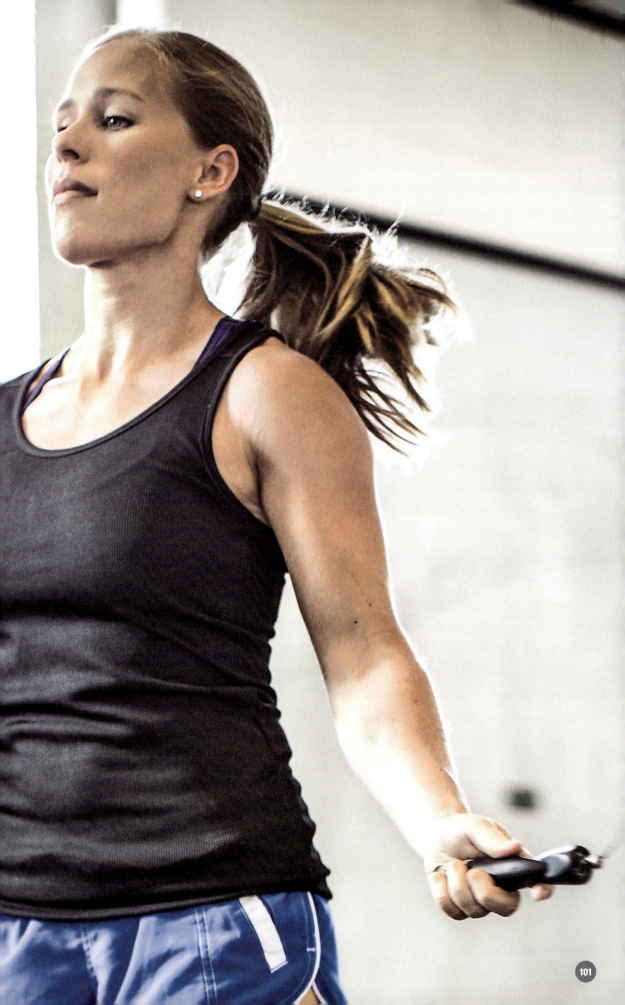

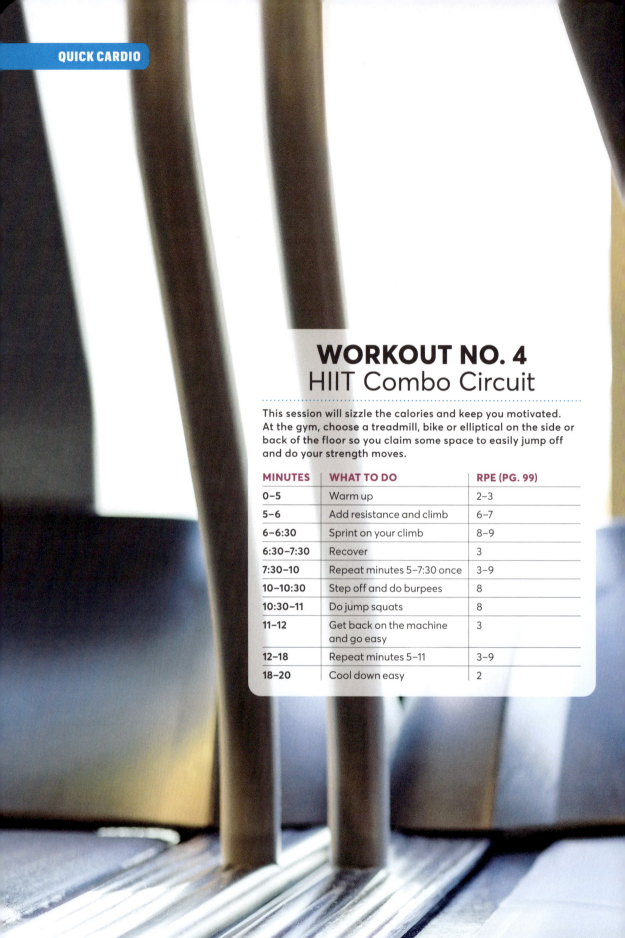

WORKOUT NO. 4
HIIT Combo Circuit

This session will sizzle the calories and keep you motivated. At the gym, choose a treadmill, bike or elliptical on the side or back of the floor so you claim some space to easily jump off and do your strength moves.

MINUTES	WHAT TO DO	RPE (PG. 99)
0–5	Warm up	2–3
5–6	Add resistance and climb	6–7
6–6:30	Sprint on your climb	8–9
6:30–7:30	Recover	3
7:30–10	Repeat minutes 5–7:30 once	3–9
10–10:30	Step off and do burpees	8
10:30–11	Do jump squats	8
11–12	Get back on the machine and go easy	3
12–18	Repeat minutes 5–11	3–9
18–20	Cool down easy	2

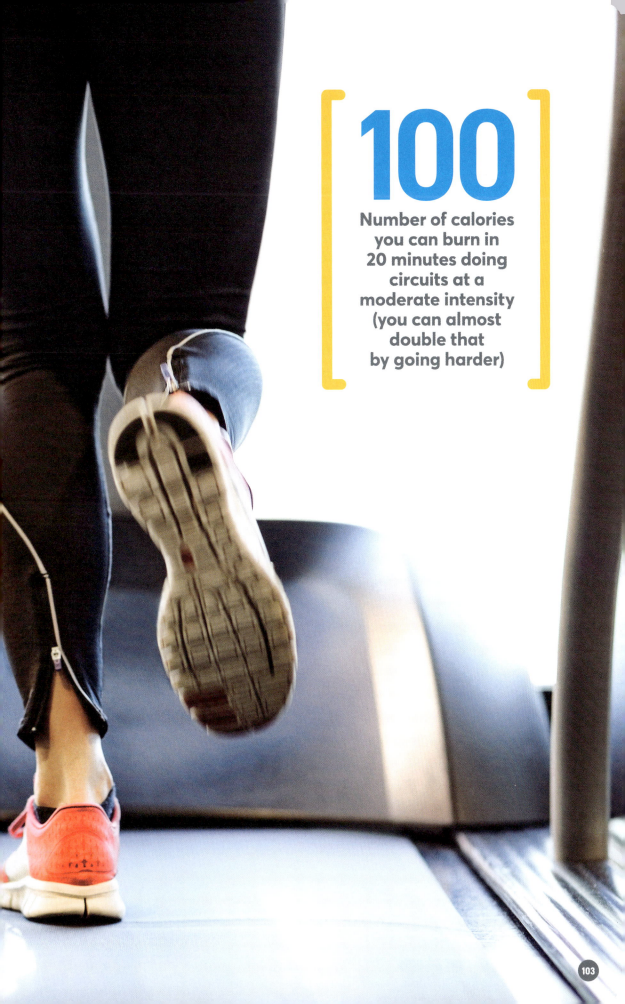

100

Number of calories you can burn in 20 minutes doing circuits at a moderate intensity (you can almost double that by going harder)

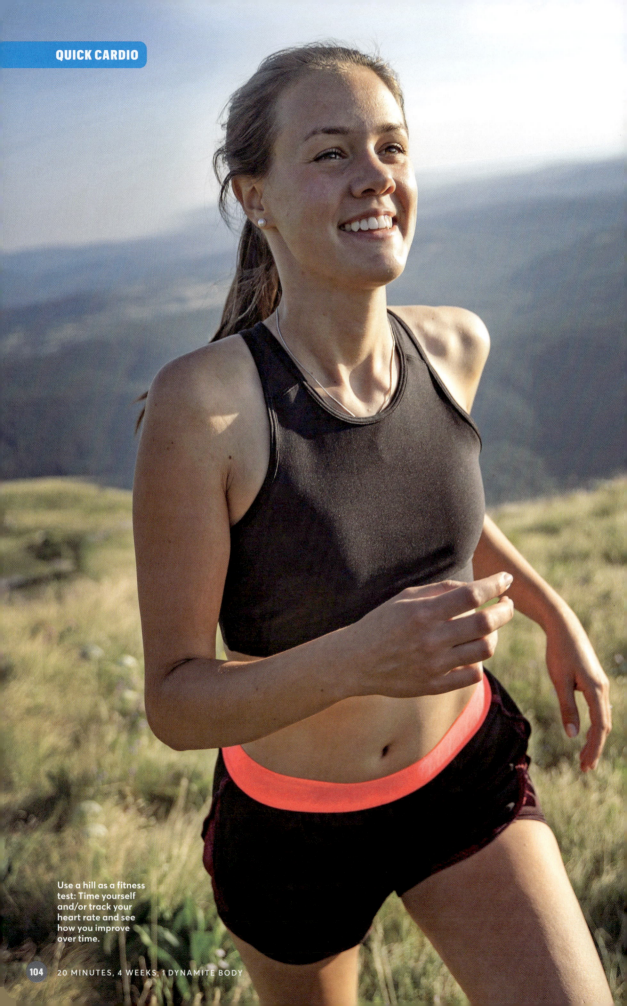

Use a hill as a fitness test: Time yourself and/or track your heart rate and see how you improve over time.

Run for the Hills

Getting fitter is a "good" uphill climb with these workouts.

You're out for a workout, you look up and there it is: the hill. Maybe you dread it, but you tackle the incline anyway. Or maybe you detour around it. Some of you might even savor the challenge and charge right up. However you approach them, hills are tough, but they're also a fantastic way to improve your strength and fitness level. "Because you're fighting against gravity (or the flywheel, if you're riding indoors on a bike), your heart rate increases, which offers a cardio bonus," says Karla Walsh, an indoor cycling instructor at CycleBar in West Des Moines, Iowa. "It's also a great mental challenge to push your body outside of its comfort zone, so your brain will score benefits, too."

You can work hills into your normal route so you hit them every so often, or you might center your entire workout on one big beast and tackle it in interval fashion: You go up, turn around and recover on the way down, then repeat. It's easier to control your hills indoors on a machine, but outdoor hills at least offer some scenery. The following workouts are designed for hiking, walking, biking and running. Just follow the time and intensity guides. Another good thing about a hill? It's easier on the other side.

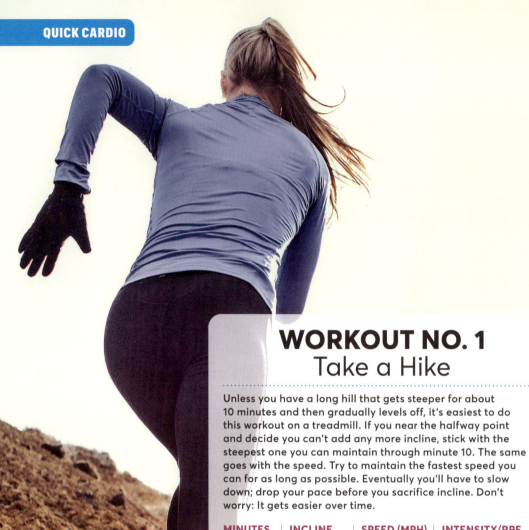

WORKOUT NO. 1
Take a Hike

Unless you have a long hill that gets steeper for about 10 minutes and then gradually levels off, it's easiest to do this workout on a treadmill. If you near the halfway point and decide you can't add any more incline, stick with the steepest one you can maintain through minute 10. The same goes with the speed. Try to maintain the fastest speed you can for as long as possible. Eventually you'll have to slow down; drop your pace before you sacrifice incline. Don't worry: It gets easier over time.

MINUTES	INCLINE	SPEED (MPH)	INTENSITY/RPE
0–1	1	3.5–3.8	Easy/2
1–2	2	3.5–3.8	Easy/2
2–3	2	3.5–3.8	Moderate/3
3–4	3	3.5–3.8	Moderate/4
4–5	4	3.5–3.8	Moderate/4
5–6	6	3.5–3.8	Moderate/5
6–7	8	3.5–3.8	Somewhat hard/7
7–8	10	3.3–3.5	Somewhat hard/7
8–9	12	3.3–3.5	Hard/8
9–10	14	3.0–3.3	Very hard/9
10–11	14	3.0–3.3	Very hard/9
11–12	12	3.3–3.5	Hard/8
12–13	11	3.3–3.5	Hard/8
13–14	10	3.3–3.5	Somewhat hard/7
14–15	8	3.5–3.8	Somewhat hard/7
15–16	6	3.5–3.8	Somewhat hard/7
16–17	4	3.5–3.8	Moderate/4
17–18	2	3.5–3.8	Moderate/3
18–19	1	3.5–3.8	Easy/2
19–20	0	3.3–3.5	Easy/2

THE DEETS

▶ **WHAT TO DO**
Once or twice a week, incorporate hills with one of the following three workouts, designed for different cardio activities.
▶ **GEAR** You'll need a cardio machine, or try it outdoors.

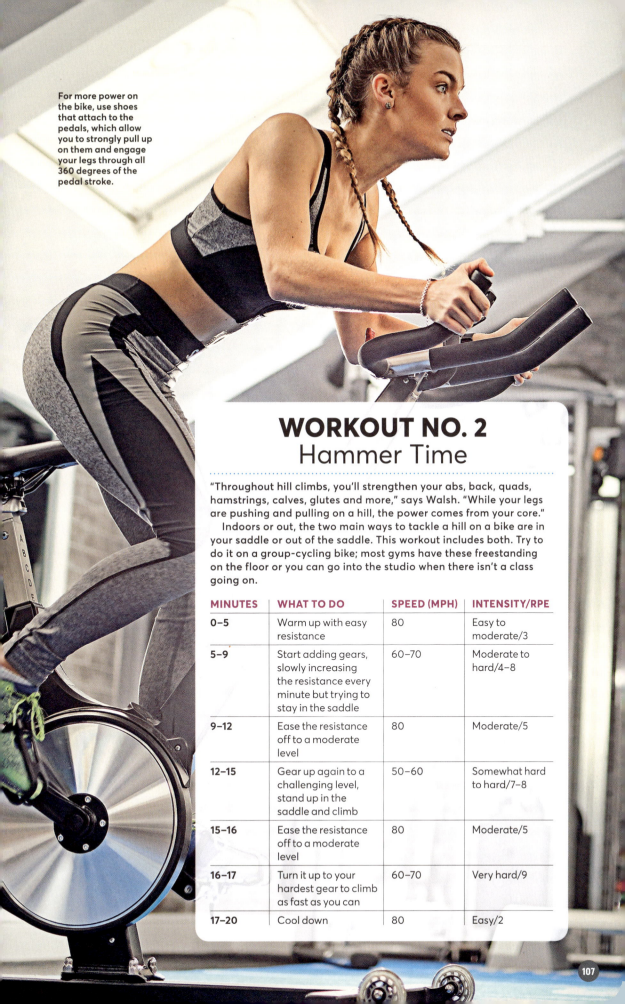

For more power on the bike, use shoes that attach to the pedals, which allow you to strongly pull up on them and engage your legs through all 360 degrees of the pedal stroke.

WORKOUT NO. 2
Hammer Time

"Throughout hill climbs, you'll strengthen your abs, back, quads, hamstrings, calves, glutes and more," says Walsh. "While your legs are pushing and pulling on a hill, the power comes from your core."

Indoors or out, the two main ways to tackle a hill on a bike are in your saddle or out of the saddle. This workout includes both. Try to do it on a group-cycling bike; most gyms have these freestanding on the floor or you can go into the studio when there isn't a class going on.

MINUTES	WHAT TO DO	SPEED (MPH)	INTENSITY/RPE
0–5	Warm up with easy resistance	80	Easy to moderate/3
5–9	Start adding gears, slowly increasing the resistance every minute but trying to stay in the saddle	60–70	Moderate to hard/4–8
9–12	Ease the resistance off to a moderate level	80	Moderate/5
12–15	Gear up again to a challenging level, stand up in the saddle and climb	50–60	Somewhat hard to hard/7–8
15–16	Ease the resistance off to a moderate level	80	Moderate/5
16–17	Turn it up to your hardest gear to climb as fast as you can	60–70	Very hard/9
17–20	Cool down	80	Easy/2

Keep your upper body relaxed—shoulders down and hands in easy fists—as you climb.

WORKOUT NO. 3
Run It Up

Outdoors you can choose a hilly route or pick just one hill that takes maybe 15 to 30 seconds to climb and do hill repeats. Indoors you have more versatility, like with this rolling hills treadmill routine. (Everyone's speed is different. Use the intensity guide to adjust your speed if what's listed is too easy/challenging.)

MINUTES	INCLINE	SPEED (MPH)	INTENSITY/RPE
0–5	0	5.5–6.0	Easy to moderate/4
5–6	3	6.0–6.5	Moderate to somewhat hard/5–7
6–7	0	6.0	Moderate/5
7–8	5	5.8–6.2	Somewhat hard/7
8–9	0	6.0	Moderate/5
9–10	7	5.5–6.0	Hard to very hard/8–9
10–11	0	6.0	Moderate/5
11–12	2	6.0–6.2	Moderate/6
12–13	3	6.0–6.2	Moderate to somewhat hard/5–7
13–14	4	5.8–6.2	Somewhat hard to hard/7–8
14–15	5	5.5–6.0	Somewhat hard to hard/7–8
15–16	6	5.5–6.0	Hard to very hard/8–9
16–17	7	5.0–5.5	Very hard/9
17–20	0	3.5	Easy/2

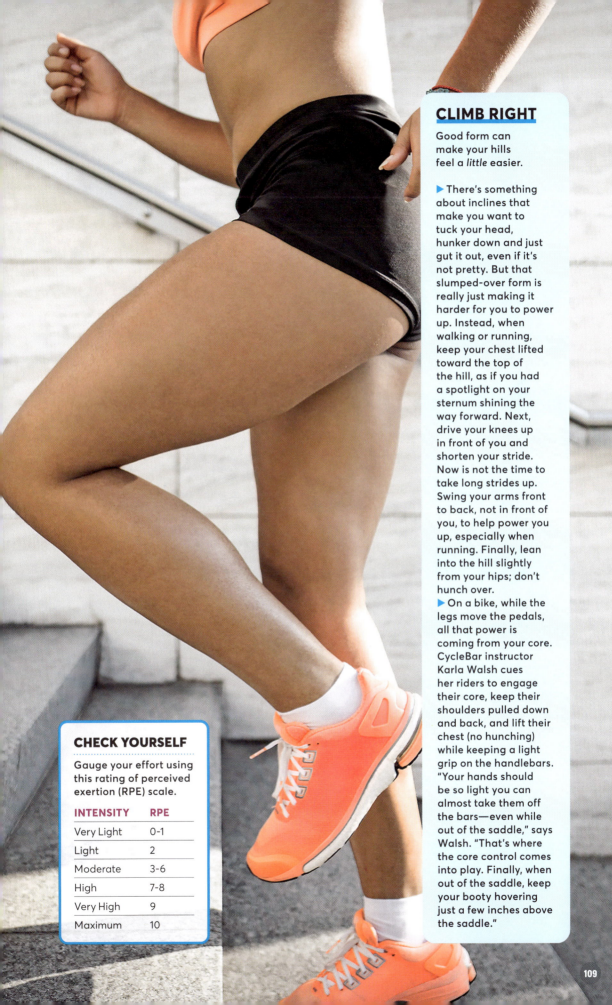

CLIMB RIGHT

Good form can make your hills feel a *little* easier.

▶ There's something about inclines that make you want to tuck your head, hunker down and just gut it out, even if it's not pretty. But that slumped-over form is really just making it harder for you to power up. Instead, when walking or running, keep your chest lifted toward the top of the hill, as if you had a spotlight on your sternum shining the way forward. Next, drive your knees up in front of you and shorten your stride. Now is not the time to take long strides up. Swing your arms front to back, not in front of you, to help power you up, especially when running. Finally, lean into the hill slightly from your hips; don't hunch over.

▶ On a bike, while the legs move the pedals, all that power is coming from your core. CycleBar instructor Karla Walsh cues her riders to engage their core, keep their shoulders pulled down and back, and lift their chest (no hunching) while keeping a light grip on the handlebars. "Your hands should be so light you can almost take them off the bars—even while out of the saddle," says Walsh. "That's where the core control comes into play. Finally, when out of the saddle, keep your booty hovering just a few inches above the saddle."

CHECK YOURSELF

Gauge your effort using this rating of perceived exertion (RPE) scale.

INTENSITY	RPE
Very Light	0-1
Light	2
Moderate	3-6
High	7-8
Very High	9
Maximum	10

HIIT It Hard

This efficient style of training ups your calorie burn during and after a session—and anyone can do it!

Back in the '80s and '90s, "cardio" meant going for a long run, walk or bike ride at an intensity that allowed you to maintain your pace for 45 minutes or longer. That could burn some serious calories, but who has the time?

Enter HIIT: high-intensity interval training. It's the ultimate workout hack and involves alternating between vigorous exercise bursts and easy recovery periods. The point is to train your body to recover quickly after exercise, which improves your fitness level. Study after study has shown that this style of training, while taking significantly less time, has similar benefits as longer bouts of exercise does. It can enhance fat-burning, improve how your body processes sugar, and also boost your heart and lungs' ability to utilize oxygen. A 2017 research review published in the *British Journal of Sports Medicine* found that HIIT performed for 12 weeks or longer reduced body fat, waist circumference, resting heart rate and blood pressure in overweight or obese subjects (much of the HIIT research has been done with people who have excess weight). If you've been trying to drop pounds and have hit a plateau, HIIT can help get the scale moving again (as long as your diet is under control).

Best of all, you don't have to be a natural-born sprinter to do it. Even cardiac rehab patients can do HIIT-style training, although it's at a much lower intensity. You go at the level that feels "intense" to you, based on your heart rate, RPE and/or the talk test (for a review of these, see page 15). Another bonus: You can utilize this style of workout with any activity, including walking, running, biking, rowing, the elliptical, stair climbing and more. You can even do it with strength or calisthenics-style moves. "It's very user-friendly and has so many benefits, including decreasing abdominal fat and revving your metabolism," says Patricia Friberg, a fitness and wellness coach in Los Angeles. "And 20 minutes is the sweet spot for HIIT training." All you need is a machine if you're not going to do it outside, a stopwatch or a smartphone app (we like the Interval Timer app). Now you're ready to HIIT it!

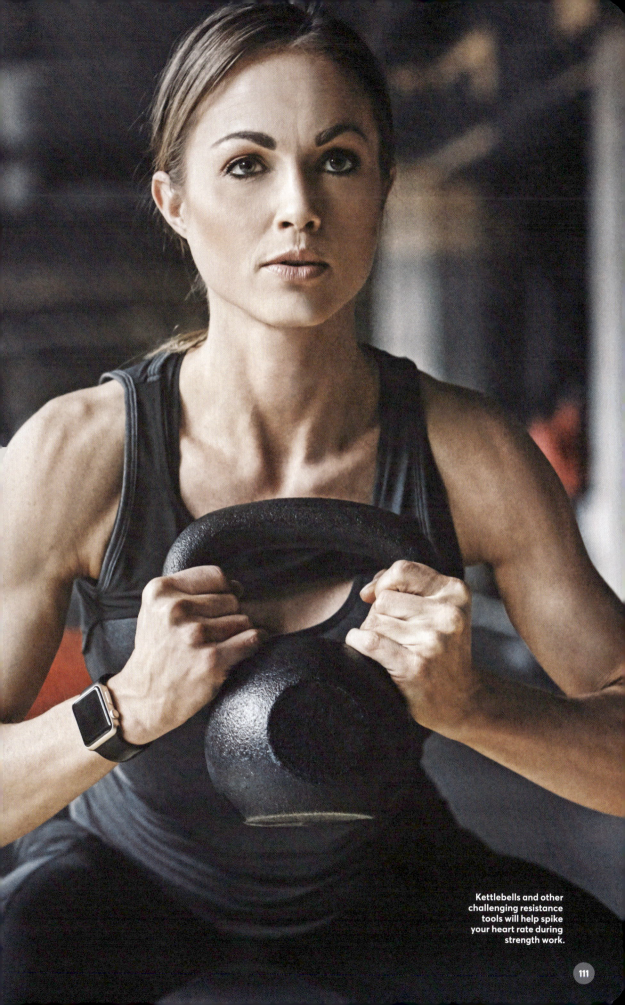

Kettlebells and other challenging resistance tools will help spike your heart rate during strength work.

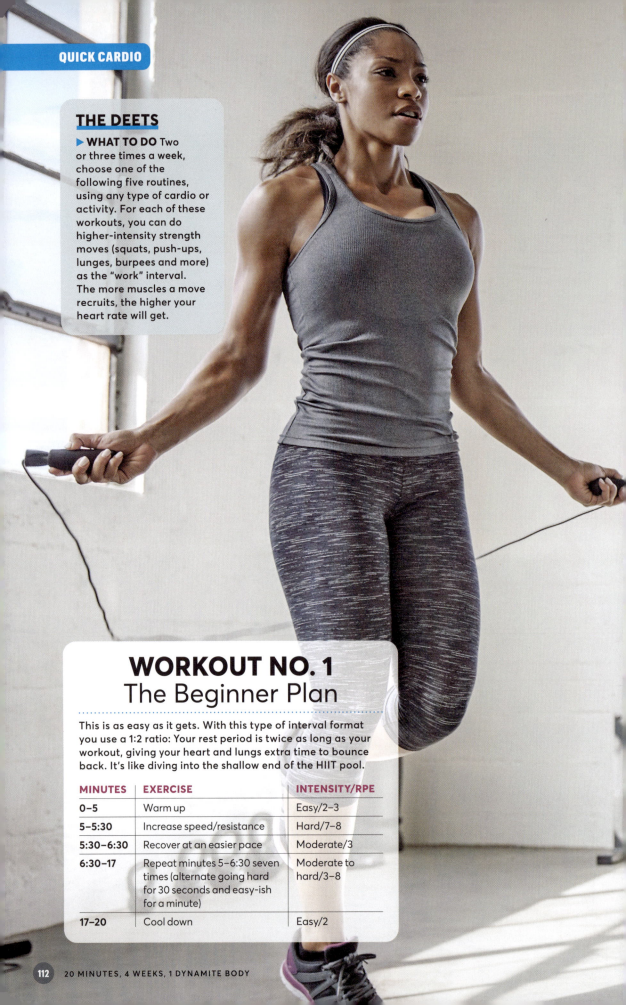

THE DEETS

▶ **WHAT TO DO** Two or three times a week, choose one of the following five routines, using any type of cardio or activity. For each of these workouts, you can do higher-intensity strength moves (squats, push-ups, lunges, burpees and more) as the "work" interval. The more muscles a move recruits, the higher your heart rate will get.

WORKOUT NO. 1
The Beginner Plan

This is as easy as it gets. With this type of interval format you use a 1:2 ratio: Your rest period is twice as long as your workout, giving your heart and lungs extra time to bounce back. It's like diving into the shallow end of the HIIT pool.

MINUTES	EXERCISE	INTENSITY/RPE
0–5	Warm up	Easy/2–3
5–5:30	Increase speed/resistance	Hard/7–8
5:30–6:30	Recover at an easier pace	Moderate/3
6:30–17	Repeat minutes 5–6:30 seven times (alternate going hard for 30 seconds and easy-ish for a minute)	Moderate to hard/3–8
17–20	Cool down	Easy/2

WORKOUT NO. 2
HIIT Your Stride

This routine involves equal work and recovery bouts (a 1:1 ratio) and gives you an extra minute of rest in the middle. Don't need it? Continue the interval format through minute 16.

MINUTES	EXERCISE	INTENSITY/RPE
0–5	Warm up	Easy/2–3
5–5:30	Increase speed/resistance	Hard/7–8
5:30–6	Recover	Moderate/3–4
6–10	Repeat minutes 5–6 four times (alternate going hard then easy-ish 30 seconds)	Moderate to hard/3–8
10–11	Go easy (extend the final recovery period)	Easy/2–3
11–16	Repeat minutes 5–6 five times	Moderate to hard/3–8
16–20	Cool down	Easy/2

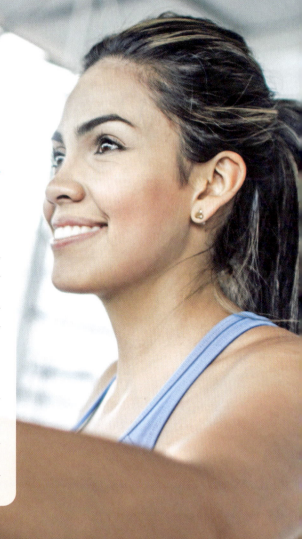

CHECK YOURSELF

Gauge your effort using this rating of perceived exertion (RPE) scale.

INTENSITY	RPE
Very Light	0-1
Light	2
Moderate	3-6
High	7-8
Very High	9
Maximum	10

WORKOUT NO. 3
The Advanced Option

Now try the more challenging style of interval, with a 2:1 work-to-recovery ratio, which means you have less time to recover.

MINUTES	EXERCISE	INTENSITY/RPE
0–5	Warm up	Easy/2–3
5–6	Increase speed/resistance	Hard/8
6–6:30	Recover	Moderate/3
6:30–17	Repeat minutes 5–6:30 seven times (alternate going hard for one minute and easy for 30 seconds)	Moderate to hard/3–8
17–20	Cool down	Easy/2

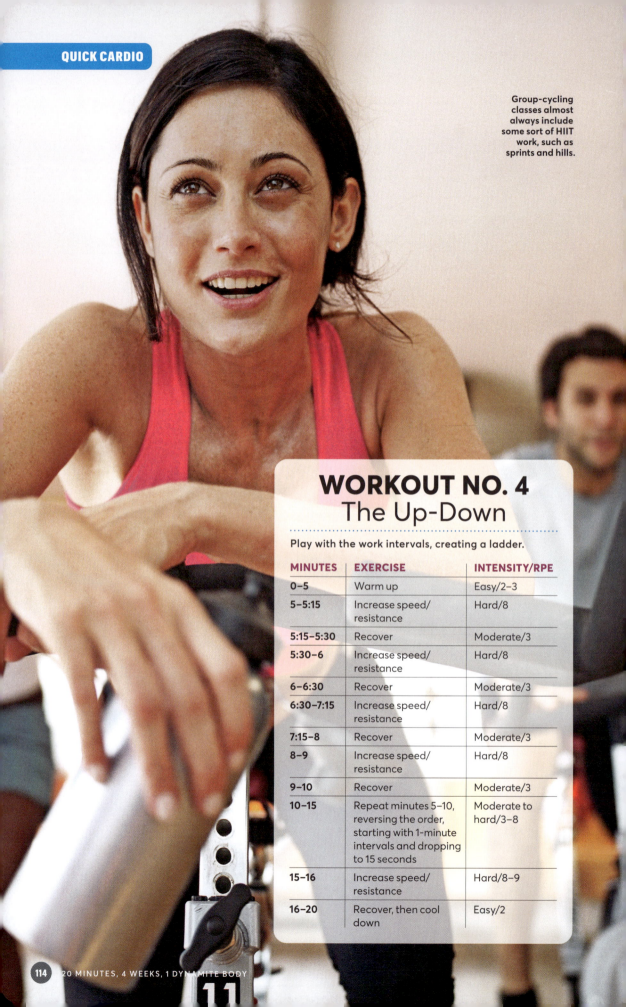

Group-cycling classes almost always include some sort of HIIT work, such as sprints and hills.

WORKOUT NO. 4
The Up-Down

Play with the work intervals, creating a ladder.

MINUTES	EXERCISE	INTENSITY/RPE
0–5	Warm up	Easy/2–3
5–5:15	Increase speed/resistance	Hard/8
5:15–5:30	Recover	Moderate/3
5:30–6	Increase speed/resistance	Hard/8
6–6:30	Recover	Moderate/3
6:30–7:15	Increase speed/resistance	Hard/8
7:15–8	Recover	Moderate/3
8–9	Increase speed/resistance	Hard/8
9–10	Recover	Moderate/3
10–15	Repeat minutes 5–10, reversing the order, starting with 1-minute intervals and dropping to 15 seconds	Moderate to hard/3–8
15–16	Increase speed/resistance	Hard/8–9
16–20	Recover, then cool down	Easy/2

WORKOUT NO. 5
Block Party

This session is divided up into three different types of intervals.

MINUTES	EXERCISE	INTENSITY/RPE
0–5	Warm up	Easy to moderate/2–3
BLOCK 1		
5–6	Increase speed/resistance	Hard/8
6–7	Recover	Moderate/3
7–11	Repeat minutes 5–7 twice	Moderate to hard/3–8
BLOCK 2		
11–11:30	Increase speed/resistance	Hard/8
11:30–12	Recover	Moderate/3
12–14	Repeat minute 11–12 twice	Moderate to hard/3–8
BLOCK 3		
14–15	Go all out for the first 15 seconds, then drop the intensity slightly every 15 seconds after that	Very hard/9–10
15–16	Recover	Moderate/3
16–18	Repeat minutes 14–16 once	Moderate to very hard/3–10
18–20	Cool down	Easy/2

THE 4-MINUTE WORKOUT

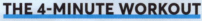

▶ **IN 1996,** researcher Izumi Tabata tested a fast, intense "workout" as part of a study comparing high-intensity interval training with regular (60-minute) moderate-intensity sessions. He found that both approaches improved aerobic capacity, but only the intervals improved anaerobic capacity (the ability to maintain a high level of effort), despite the drastic difference in time spent exercising.
▶ **HERE'S HOW** a Tabata routine works: After a brief warm-up, you go all out (as hard as you can) for 20 seconds, then rest for 10 seconds. Repeat that pattern for a total of 8 rounds, then cool down easy.

If you're doing it right, you'll be pretty miserable during those 20-second bursts; they're that hard. In the lab, study subjects typically do Tabata intervals on a special type of stationary bike that incorporates your arms and legs, but you can use any type. It won't feel good, but it's over in 4 minutes!

Boot Camp Blast

Use this workout to burn serious calories while working your entire body.

You don't need a treadmill or bike to get a good cardio workout. Using your own body weight, and especially those large energy-guzzling muscles in your core, hips and legs, you can work up a sweat, burning up to 10 calories a minute (the equivalent of an easy running pace). The bonus: You can do it anywhere you have a little space to move around. Don't have 20 minutes to spare? Just do it for 10 (or fewer), as a way to torch calories and spike your metabolism throughout the day.

This workout is plyo-heavy, meaning there are a lot of moves that involve jumping and hopping. If you're not quite up to this, keep the jumps and hops very low or just take them out and step side to side or back and forth. If you need more rest between the exercises, take out the skipping and pause for 30 seconds, then move on to the next exercise.

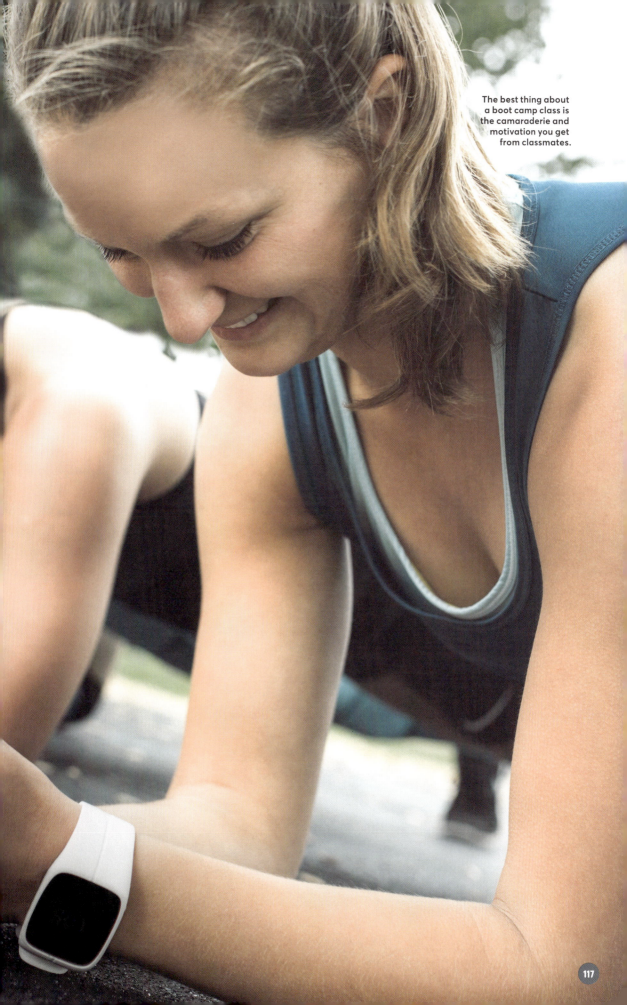

The best thing about a boot camp class is the camaraderie and motivation you get from classmates.

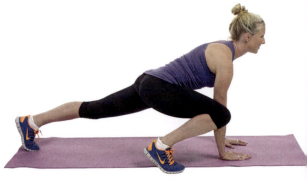

THE DEETS

▶ **WHAT TO DO** Perform each move for 30 seconds in order, without resting. After the last move, rest for a minute, then repeat the circuit once more.
▶ **GEAR** Just a mat for comfort.
▶ **GET STARTED** Warm up for 5 minutes beforehand then cool down for a few minutes afterward with some easy stretching (see page 134).

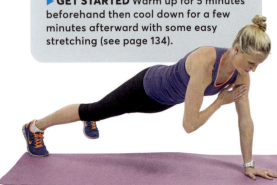

❶ PLANK TAP

▶ **Works core**
Get in high plank position on hands and toes so body is straight from head to heels. Keeping the rest of your body as still as possible, tap left shoulder with right hand [shown], then right shoulder with left hand. Continue back and forth for 30 seconds. (You'll do this again in move No. 7.)

❷ SKIPPING

▶ **Works legs and core**
Stand with feet hip-width apart and arms at your sides, elbows slightly bent as if you were holding an end of a jump rope in each hand [not shown]. Start twirling the imaginary rope as you raise one knee and then the other to skip over it. (If it's easier, just hop over the "rope" with feet together.) Continue for 30 seconds. Come back to this after each move.

DO THIS BETWEEN EACH MOVE

> **"Discipline is the bridge between goals and accomplishment."**
> —JIM ROHN, ENTREPRENEUR

❸ WIDE-LEG MOUNTAIN CLIMBER

▶ **Works glutes and core**
Get in high plank position on the floor with wrists aligned under shoulders and body straight from head to heels. Draw right leg outside right elbow [shown]. Step back and switch legs. As you get the hang of it, hop feet forward and back. Keep core engaged the entire time. Continue for 30 seconds, then return to skipping.

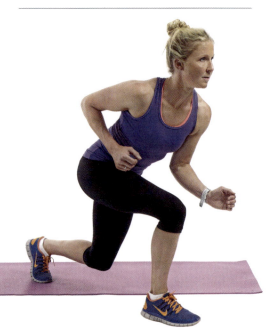

❹ FRONT-TO-BACK SPRINT

▶ **Works legs, glutes and core**
Stand with feet hip-width apart and arms at sides. Squat, staying low with your knees bent. Take two steps forward [shown] and touch the ground with the opposite arm of the forward leg (if right leg is in front, touch left hand to floor). Reverse, taking two steps back to the starting position and touching the floor, then repeat, leading with the opposite leg. Continue for 30 seconds, staying low. Once you get the feel for it, speed up your steps. Continue for 30 seconds, then return to skipping.

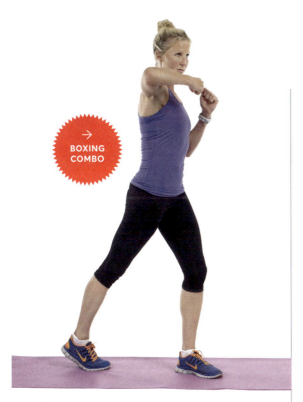

BOXING COMBO →

⑤ SPARRING

▶ **Works legs, core and arms**
Stand with left foot in front of right. Punch forward (jab) with left arm, then right (cross). Next, bend right elbow, lift it so it's parallel to the floor and draw it around in front of you, as if hitting a bag with it [shown]. Continue for 30 seconds, then switch stance and arms and repeat for 30 seconds. Return to skipping.

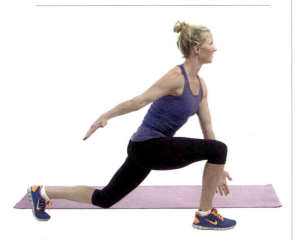

⑥ PLYO LUNGE

▶ **Works legs, glutes and core**
Stand with feet hip-width apart then lunge forward with right leg, lowering left knee almost to the floor. Reach left arm forward, with your right arm back or to the side [shown]. From here, spring up, switching arms and legs. (If this is too hard, step right foot back and lunge forward with left leg.) Continue, alternating legs, for 30 seconds, then return to skipping.

⑦ BURPEES

▶ **Works entire body**
Stand with feet hip-width apart. Squat low, placing hands on the floor in front of knees, then hop or step feet back so you're in a high plank position. Tap right shoulder with left hand, then switch sides. (Add a push-up here for more of a challenge.) Jump or step feet toward hands again, then spring straight up, reaching arms overhead [shown]. Continue for 30 seconds, then return to skipping.

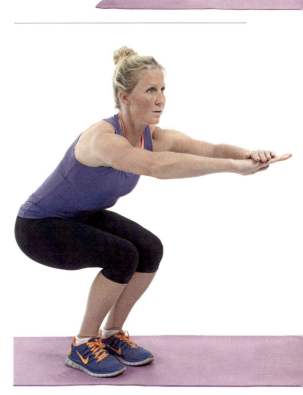

⑧ OUT-IN SQUAT JUMP

▶ **Works legs and glutes**
Stand with feet hip-width apart and squat low, extending arms in front of you, one hand on top of the other. Maintaining low-squat position, hop feet wide, keeping knees aligned over feet, then hop feet together [shown]. Continue for 30 seconds, then return to skipping before resting.

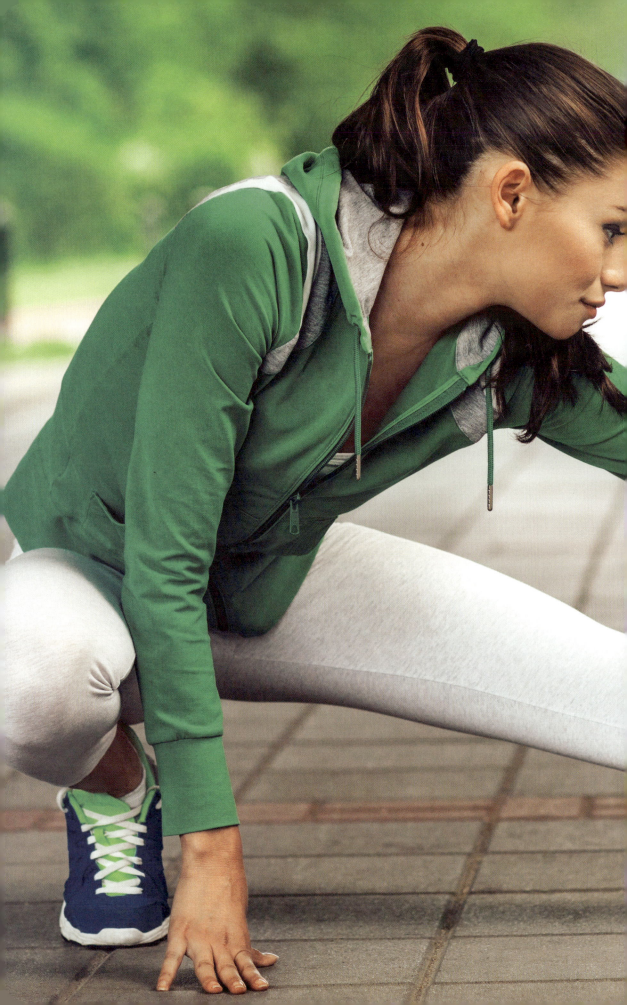

FEEL-GOOD STRETCHES

↓

Limber Up

THE UNSUNG HERO OF FITNESS, FLEXIBILITY EXERCISES ENHANCE YOUR RANGE OF MOTION AND PROVIDE YOU WITH AN EXCELLENT OPPORTUNITY TO CHECK IN WITH YOUR BODY IN A MORE MINDFUL WAY.

Yoga Flow

Up the aerobic challenge of your poses with this variation on a classic sequence.

The words "yoga" and "cardio" would seem to be at opposite ends of the exercise and heart rate spectrums. For many yoga styles, that's true. You might burn the equivalent of a walk, but when you start flowing quickly from pose to pose—matching movements with your breath—your heart rate rises and you can burn several hundred calories an hour, comparable to riding a bike or jogging. But you gotta *move*. Hot yoga might get your heart rate up simply because it's like a sauna in there; you're holding the poses, not flowing. Vinyasa yoga, where you're moving fluidly from pose to pose, is the cardio queen in yoga.

Vinyasa style or not, many yoga classes start with a series of moves called *surya namaskara* A and B (aka sun salutations), which are meant to warm up the body. It's like saying,

"Oh, hey there, body. How are you today?" "Sun salutations move the body in different directions; there's flexion and extension, so it's preparing you physically and energetically," says Diane Malaspina, e-RYT, a psychologist and yoga instructor in Virginia Beach, Virginia. "If you move quickly you can increase your heart rate and get an energy boost, but there's also this meditative quality that comes from linking the movements with the breath."

The flow on the following pages is a variation on the classic Sun Salutation series. You'll go through Series A on its own a few times first, and then add on with Series B poses. There are a few poses in the series that you hold for several breaths (like isometrics), which is more challenging than it might seem. You'll finish with a few held poses before settling in to savasana. Hit the mat, everyone!

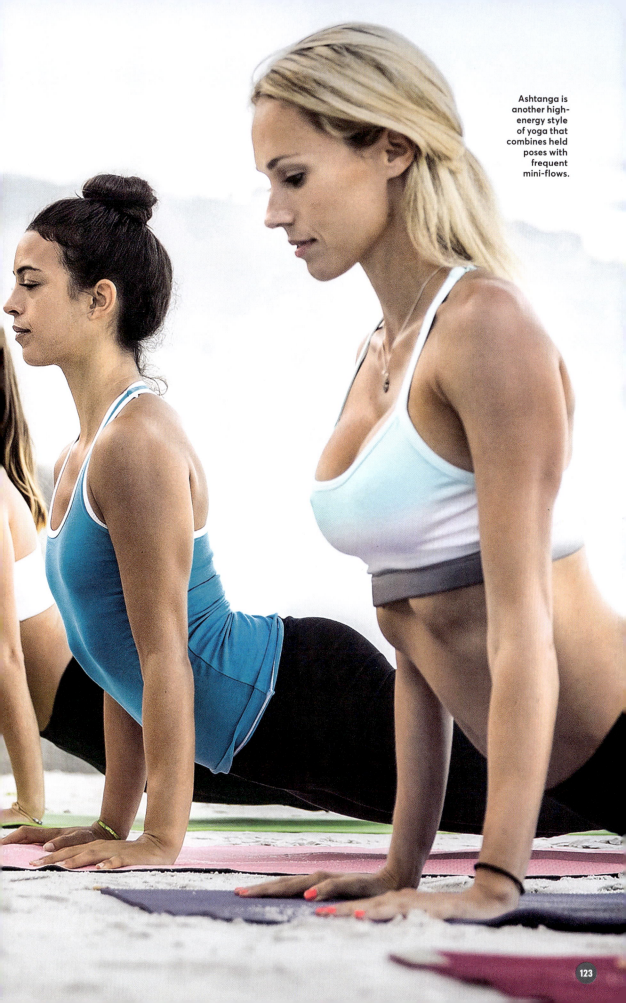

Ashtanga is another high-energy style of yoga that combines held poses with frequent mini-flows.

SERIES A HERE COMES THE SUN

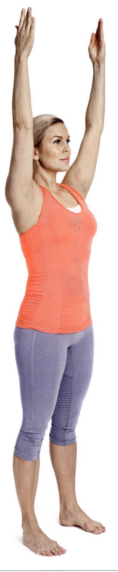

❶ EXTENDED MOUNTAIN POSE
(*TADASANA URDHVA HASTASANA*)

Stand with feet hip-width apart, arms at sides with palms facing forward. Try to create length from head to toe, grounding down through the feet as you lift the top of your head toward the ceiling. Draw your shoulder blades down and open through the chest. Take a few breaths here and once you feel grounded and calm, start the flow by inhaling and raising your arms wide out to the sides and overhead, palms facing each other [shown].

❷ CHAIR POSE
(*UTKATASANA*)

Keeping your arms overhead and even with your ears, exhale as you shift your hips back as if you were going to sit in a chair behind you [shown]. Knees stay parallel (feet and knees can be closer together, which is more challenging). Hold for 3 breaths.

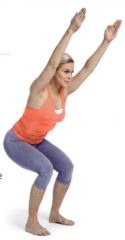

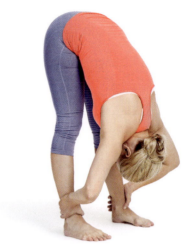

❸ STANDING FORWARD FOLD
(*UTTANASANA*)

On an exhale, bend over and place your hands on the floor or hold onto your ankles [shown]. Let your head sink toward the floor.

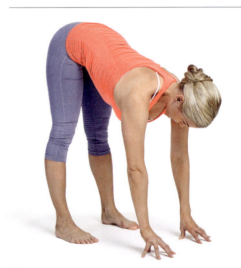

❹ HALF FORWARD FOLD
(*ARDHA UTTANASANA*)

Inhale as you straighten your spine and rise halfway up, fingertips grazing the floor [shown] or on your shins.

❺ STANDING FORWARD FOLD
(*UTTANASANA*)

Exhale and fold all the way over (see #3), head reaching for the floor (knees can stay bent).

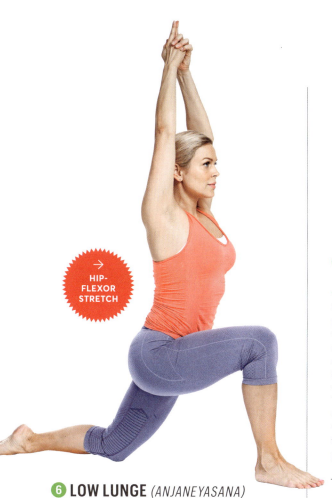

HIP-FLEXOR STRETCH →

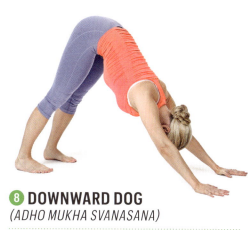

8 DOWNWARD DOG
(ADHO MUKHA SVANASANA)

Exhale as you lift hips into an inverted-V position [shown]. Press hands into the mat as you widen your fingers, draw your shoulders away from your ears and contract the quadriceps muscles at the front of your thighs. (Your heels don't have to touch the mat.) Let your head hang heavy, lengthening your spine. Take 5 breaths here. Reverse the series, skipping Cobra, to return to Mountain pose (step forward with left leg into Low Lunge). Repeat Series A twice more, then continue to Series B (turn the page) from Downward Dog.

6 LOW LUNGE *(ANJANEYASANA)*

Inhale as you step your left leg back and come into a deep lunge, left knee on the floor. Bring your arms overhead, clasping hands and extending your index fingers. (Keep arms parallel if that's more comfortable.) Front knee should be aligned over front ankle [shown]. Exhale as you place hands on either side of your front foot and step back into plank position, body straight from head to heels [not shown]; slowly lower yourself all the way down to the mat, keeping your elbows at your sides and hands near your chest.

TAKE IT OFF THE MAT

▶ You can use the flow here as its own quickie cardio session, as a warm-up before a strength workout (minus the last four poses) or for recovery on an off day. (Adjust the number of times through to fit the time you have available). Play around to see what works to liven up your routine and kick up your calorie count.

7 COBRA POSE *(BHUJANGASANA)*

Inhale as you lift your head and chest off the mat, keeping your neck long (don't look up or down; gaze slightly forward). Legs and hips are on the mat, toes pointed [shown]. Exhale as you lower your head to the mat. Repeat twice, then inhale as you press back up to plank.

CHEST AND AB STRETCH ↓

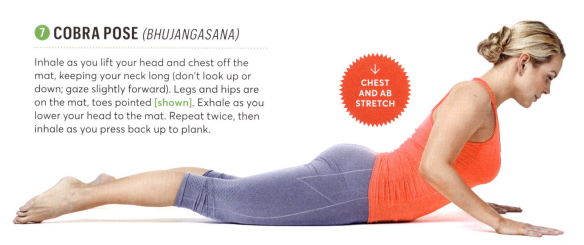

SERIES B IT'S GETTING HOT IN HERE

1 DOWNWARD DOG SPLITS
(EKA PADA ADHO MUKHA SVANASANA)

On an inhale, raise right leg behind you [shown].

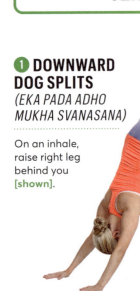

THE ULTIMATE POWER POSE

2 KNEE TO NOSE PLANK
(PHALAKASANA VARIATION)

Exhale as you shift your weight forward into a plank pose, drawing right knee toward your nose [shown]. Repeat Downward Dog Splits and flow to Knee to Nose Plank once more.

3 DOWNWARD DOG SPLITS
(EKA PADA ADHO MUKHA SVANASANA)

Inhale as you raise right leg up behind you again (aka "three-legged dog") [shown].

4 WARRIOR II POSE
(VIRABHADRASANA II)

Exhale as you look forward and step your right foot inside the right hand; lower left foot to the mat and turn left toes out 45 degrees. Inhale as you rise up and extend your arms out to each side over legs, fingers reaching to the front and back [shown]. If you look down, it's as if you're on a tightrope; a line from your front heel would bisect the instep of your back foot. Look over your front (right) arm as you draw your shoulders away from your ears and imagine pressing down on two large balloons. Keep your front knee tracking over your ankle and feel your hips opening. Take a breath or two here.

5 REVERSE WARRIOR POSE
(VIPARITA VIRABHADRASANA)

On an inhale, keep your legs stationary as you bend back over your left leg, extending right arm overhead [shown].

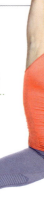
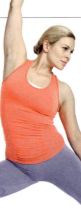

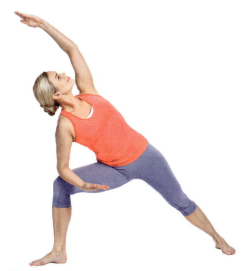

6 EXTENDED SIDE ANGLE POSE
(PARSVAKONASANA)

Exhale as you lean over right leg, placing forearm on your thigh, palm turned up, and reaching left arm overhead. Look up at your top arm [shown]. Repeat Reverse Warrior Pose and Extended Side Angle Pose twice more.

7 FLOWING HALF SQUAT
(SAHAJA ARDHA MALASANA)

On an exhale, bend over from hips and place hands on floor. Inhale as you bend right knee and sweep hands toward right foot [A]. Exhale as you shift weight to left, bending left knee and sweeping arms toward left foot [B]. Continue side to side for three more inhales and exhales. Come back to center and rise up on an inhale.

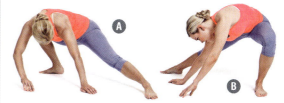

8 MOUNTAIN POSE (TADASANA)

Exhale as you step feet hip-width apart, arms at your sides [not shown]. Repeat entire series starting with Series A, leading with the left side. Do the full sequence twice on each side.

THE BIG FINISH TAKE IT TO THE FLOOR

1 CRESCENT POSE
(ALANASANA)

From Mountain Pose, inhale, arms over head, palms facing each other, as you raise your right knee up to hip height in front of you. Exhale as you step back, lowering into a lunge, back knee off the ground [shown]. Hold for 2 breaths, then step right foot forward to Mountain Pose and switch legs, stepping back with left leg. Hold for 2 breaths, then return to Mountain Pose.

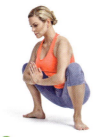

2 GARLAND POSE
(MALASANA)

From Mountain Pose, step feet shoulder-width apart, toes turned out, place palms together in front of chest and squat deep. Press upper arms against knees [shown]. Reach your tailbone toward the floor and draw shoulders down as you lift your sternum toward the ceiling. Hold for 5 breaths.

3 CHILD'S POSE
(BALASANA)

Place hands on mat and come to all fours, wrists aligned under shoulders and knees under hips. From here, sit hips back on your heels and extend arms in front of you, palms down [shown above]. Walk hands to left side, keeping right hip anchored down, and hold for 3 to 5 breaths. Repeat to the right side. Walk hands back to center and sit up.

4 CORPSE POSE
(SAVASANA)

If you're doing this as a mini-workout, you can finish lying flat on your back, arms at your sides with palms turned up [shown below]. Relax your breathing and release any remaining tension in your body, including tension in your neck, shoulders, belly, hips and ankles. Relax here for a few minutes.

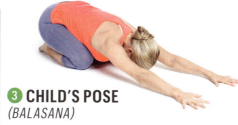

Strong
to the
Core

The mindfulness and body awareness required in yoga help you zero in on your midsection.

Yoga is an amazingly well-rounded workout: It boosts flexibility and strength, can burn serious calories, enhances mindfulness and eases stress. It's a diverse practice that doesn't stop when you step off your mat, but when you *are* on your mat, it allows you a way to be fully in your body, almost like a child discovering every inch of this skin suit that we're blessed with. You bend, twist, balance, lunge, bind and more, and as a result, it's also a fantastic workout for the core. In addition, the breath work that you do in yoga taps some of the core muscles that help stabilize your spine and torso. The next time you want a quick, crunch-less, mindful core workout—or maybe a powerful finish to a cardio session, try the following moves. Just warm up with 3 to 5 rounds of the Series A moves on pages 124 and 125, then do each of the following poses once. Om-my, what great abs you'll have!

In poses like Warrior II, you're engaging the abs to help lengthen and stabilize the spine.

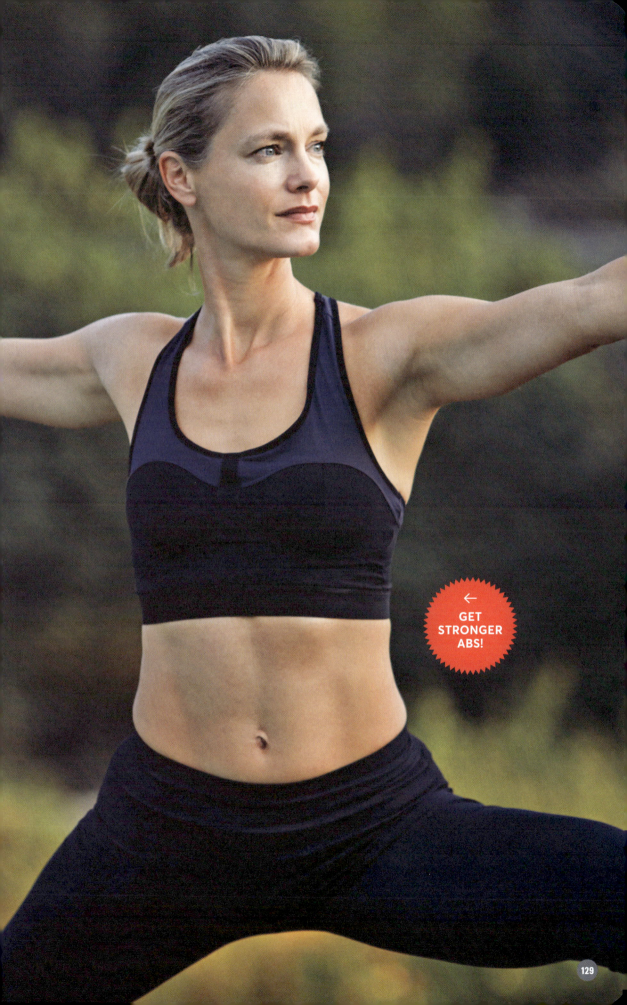

GET STRONGER ABS!

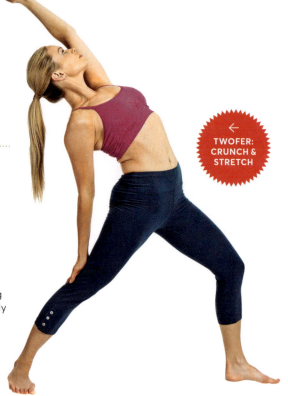

TWOFER: CRUNCH & STRETCH

① REVERSE WARRIOR POSE
(VIPARITA VIRABHADRASANA)

▶ **Works obliques and legs**

Stand with feet together, hands at sides. Step right foot back about 3 feet and turn toes out 45 to 90 degrees. Bend left knee so it's aligned over ankle and extend arms over legs, palms down (Warrior II Pose). Keeping lower body stationary (left knee stays bent), lift left arm up and overhead as you lean back over right leg, opening the left side of your body long (turn it into a gentle backbend by lifting your chest up to the ceiling slightly) **[shown]**. Hold for 5 breaths, consciously engaging the muscles on the right side of your torso. Move to Extended Side Angle.

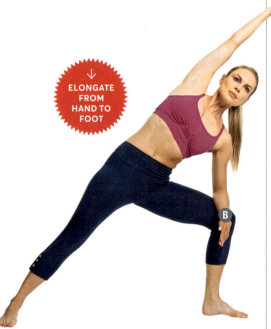

ELONGATE FROM HAND TO FOOT

② EXTENDED SIDE ANGLE POSE
(PARSVAKONASANA)

▶ **Works obliques and legs**

From Reverse Warrior, use your abs to bend over front (left) leg. Rest left forearm on thigh and extend right arm overhead, palm turned down **[shown]**. Hold here for 5 breaths. Rise back up to Warrior 2, then switch direction of legs (bend right knee) and repeat Reverse Warrior before moving into Extended Side Angle.

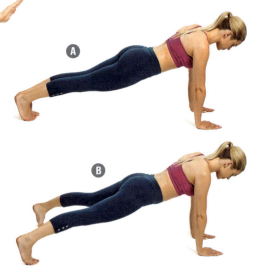

③ PLANK WITH TOE TAPS
(PHALAKASANA VARIATION)

▶ **Works entire core**

Get in high plank position on hands and toes, body straight from head to heels **[A]**. Look down, without tucking your chin, so your spine is long. Press away from the mat and press your heels behind you. Step left foot out to left, and right foot out to right, so feet are wide **[B]**; step back to center to complete 1 rep. Do 10 to 20 reps, then rest on all fours. Repeat twice, breathing evenly and deeply. Start with fewer taps and sets if this is too challenging; to make it harder, jump feet wide and then back to center.

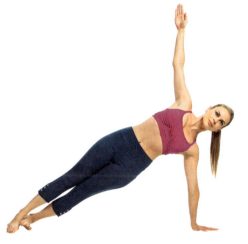

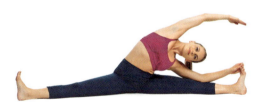

④ SIDE PLANK POSE
(VASISTHASANA)

▶ **Works entire core and glutes**

From plank position on hands and toes, lift right hand straight up and turn to right so you're balancing on left hand and outside of left foot. Shoulders should be stacked over left wrist [shown]. Hold for up to 5 breaths, then switch sides. If this is too hard, rest right foot on floor in front of left leg. For more of a challenge, pulse hips higher 10 times.

⑤ WIDE-LEG SIDE STRETCH
(PARSVA UPAVISTHA KONASANA)

▶ **Works obliques**

Sit tall with legs wide and feet flexed. Inhale as you extend arms overhead, palms facing each other and shoulders drawn down. Try to grow even taller, then exhale and use your abs to lean over left leg, reaching for left toes [shown], shin or ankle. Keep front of torso facing forward; don't turn chest toward leg. Hold for 5 breaths, then sit up and repeat to the other side.

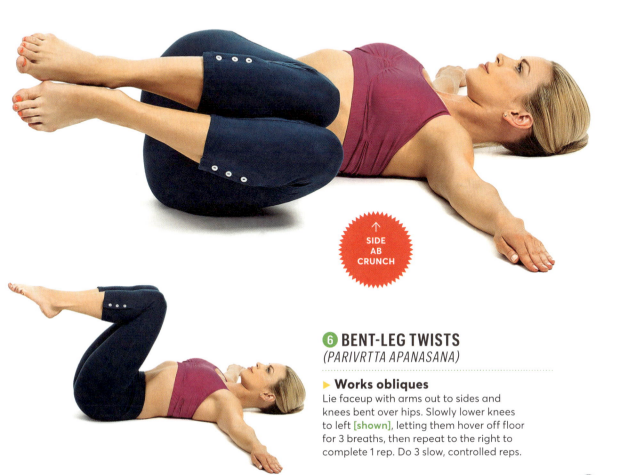

↑
SIDE
AB
CRUNCH

⑥ BENT-LEG TWISTS
(PARIVRTTA APANASANA)

▶ **Works obliques**

Lie faceup with arms out to sides and knees bent over hips. Slowly lower knees to left [shown], letting them hover off floor for 3 breaths, then repeat to the right to complete 1 rep. Do 3 slow, controlled reps.

BELLY TALK

What does it really mean to "engage your core?" It's an important concept because it's not about sucking your belly in to look slimmer; it's about creating more stability for your spine. Here are three quick ways to boost your ab awareness while creating a more stable midsection in yoga class.

▶ **DIRECTION** *Engage your "deep abs."* This means activating your transverse abdominis muscle, which is the deepest layer of your abs. You do that by drawing your belly button in slightly, like what happens if you have to cough.

▶ **DIRECTION** *Pull your bottom ribs toward your hip bones.* If engaging your transverse abs doesn't quite work for you, think of drawing your rib cage toward your pelvis. Anytime you feel like you're arching back too much and sticking your backside out, you can turn on your abs with this adjustment and take some of the stress out of the spine.

▶ **DIRECTION** *Lift your pelvic floor.* When you're trying to stop the flow of urine, you engage these pelvic muscles and the same goes in yoga. You draw them in and up.

▶ **DIRECTION** *Breathe into your entire torso.* Instead of chest breathing or just pooching out your belly with each inhale, this way of breathing expands your torso 360 degrees; your ribs will widen out to the sides and back.

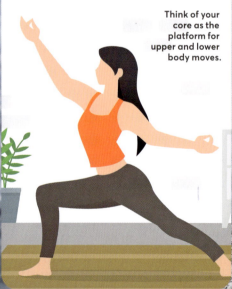

Think of your core as the platform for upper and lower body moves.

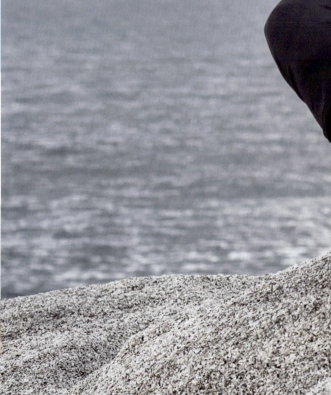

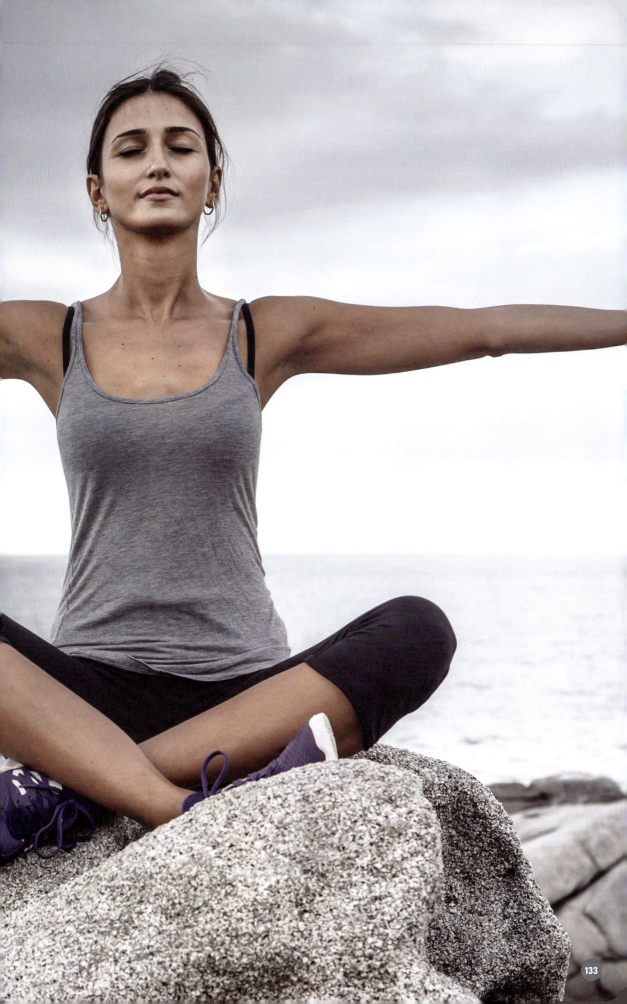

Stretch Goals

You don't have to do yoga to appreciate the effects of a gentle flexibility session for both mind and body.

It's probably the most overlooked part of your workout routine, whether due to time, boredom or just not understanding (and appreciating) its benefits, but stretching is the icing on your exercise cake. It helps preserve and enhance range of motion, which can decline with age. It can also potentially improve performance (although too much flexibility can sometimes *decrease* performance). The benefit that might be most relevant to you is that it can help work out muscle tightness and chronic contraction as a result of holding the same position for too long, such as sitting in front of a computer all day.

The stretches on the following pages target the entire body, so they're perfect after any workout. The key word here is *after*. There are a variety of stretching approaches, but the standard grab-and-hold method is best when your muscles are warm. If you prefer to stretch before a session, do it *after* you've warmed up for 5 to 10 minutes.

Some research has found that stretching between weight sets may boost muscle gains.

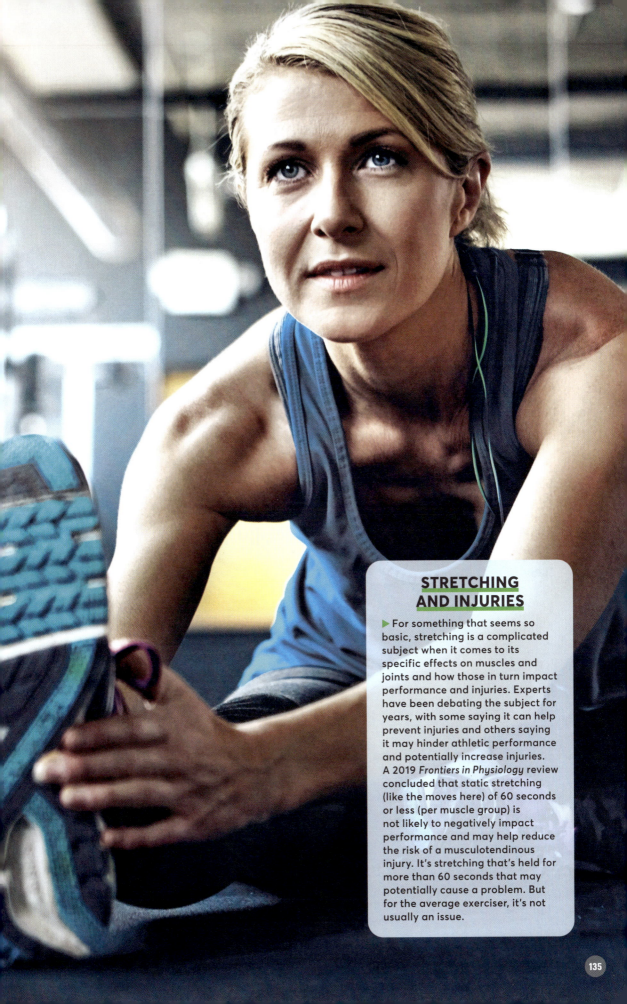

STRETCHING AND INJURIES

▶ For something that seems so basic, stretching is a complicated subject when it comes to its specific effects on muscles and joints and how those in turn impact performance and injuries. Experts have been debating the subject for years, with some saying it can help prevent injuries and others saying it may hinder athletic performance and potentially increase injuries. A 2019 *Frontiers in Physiology* review concluded that static stretching (like the moves here) of 60 seconds or less (per muscle group) is not likely to negatively impact performance and may help reduce the risk of a musculotendinous injury. It's stretching that's held for more than 60 seconds that may potentially cause a problem. But for the average exerciser, it's not usually an issue.

① STANDING QUAD STRETCH

▶ **Targets front of hip and thigh**
Stand with feet hip-width apart and bend right knee, drawing right foot up behind you. Grasp foot with right hand as you stand tall with abs engaged. Keep your right knee pointing toward the floor and even with the left leg, making sure your lower leg doesn't angle out to the side; it should be directly behind you [shown]. For more of a stretch, contract the right glute. Hold for 30 seconds, breathing deeply, then switch legs and repeat.

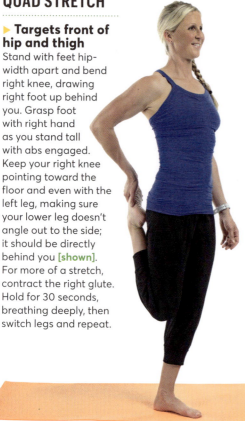

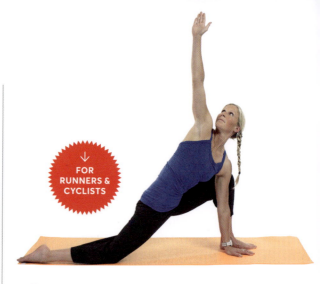

FOR RUNNERS & CYCLISTS

③ LUNGE AND TWIST

▶ **Targets front of hip and leg, chest and shoulder**
Lunge forward with left leg, knee aligned over ankle, and rest right knee on the floor. Place both hands on floor inside left foot and let the hips sink toward the floor. Contract right side glute to increase the stretch. Hold here for 30 seconds, then keep left hand on floor and twist up to right, raising right hand toward ceiling and opening chest to the side [shown]. Hold for 30 seconds, breathing deeply. Come back to all fours and sit hips back on heels for 30 seconds. Switch legs and repeat.

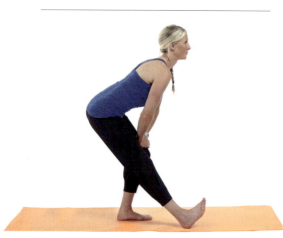

② HAMSTRING STRETCH

▶ **Targets back of upper and lower leg**
Stand with feet hip-width apart and squat about halfway. Extend right leg in front of you, toes up and heel on the floor. Keeping your back straight, squat a little deeper until you feel a stretch through the back of the right leg [shown]. Draw the toes toward you to increase the stretch. Hold for 30 seconds, breathing deeply, then switch legs and repeat.

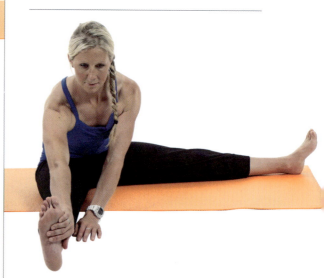

④ WIDE V STRETCH

▶ **Targets inner thigh and back of leg**
Sit tall with legs wide. Turn to face right leg and hinge forward from the hip over the leg. When you can't reach any farther forward, then round your back over your leg, resting your hands on your lower shin or grasping your foot [shown]. (Add a side stretch by reaching over leg with opposite arm.) Hold for 30 seconds, breathing deeply, then rise up, twist to the left and repeat the stretch on that side.

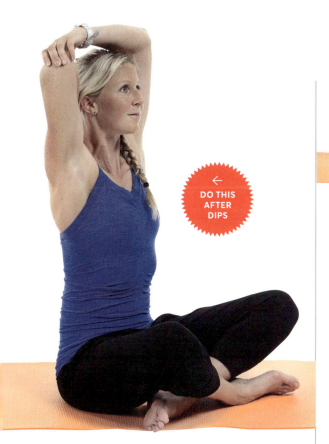

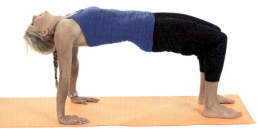

← DO THIS AFTER DIPS

7 REVERSE TABLETOP

▶ **Targets abs, hips, chest, shoulders and front of arms**

Sit with knees bent and feet flat on floor, hip-width apart. Place hands on either side of hips and slightly behind you, fingers pointing forward (if this is uncomfortable, you can turn the fingers out to the sides slightly). Lift hips so body is straight from chest to knees. Your knees should be aligned over ankles and shoulders over wrists. You may have to lower hips and adjust to find this position. You can look up at the ceiling [shown] or, if that hurts your neck, look forward. Hold for five breaths, then lower to the floor. Rest for a few breaths, then repeat once or twice.

5 TRICEPS STRETCH

▶ **Targets back of upper arm and back**

Sit tall with legs crossed (or take whatever comfortable seated position you like with hips grounded firmly on the floor). Extend right arm overhead, next to ear, and bend right elbow so right hand rests at base of neck. Grasp right elbow with left hand, drawing elbow slightly to left [shown]. Hold for 30 seconds, then switch arms and repeat.

8 LOW BACK TWIST

▶ **Targets hip and back**

Lie faceup and draw knees into chest. Grab shins and gently roll around, giving yourself a self-massage. Next, extend arms out to sides, palms down, and slowly draw knees over to right side as you look left [not shown]. Let knees rest on floor and hold the stretch for 30 seconds, breathing deeply; switch sides and repeat.

6 SUPINE FIGURE 4

▶ **Targets outer hip**

Lie faceup with knees bent and feet flat on floor. Cross left ankle over right knee, as if you were sitting in a chair, then place hands on either side of right thigh and draw it toward you, trying to keep left knee pointing out to the side (away from chest) [shown]. Hold for 30 seconds, breathing deeply, then switch legs.

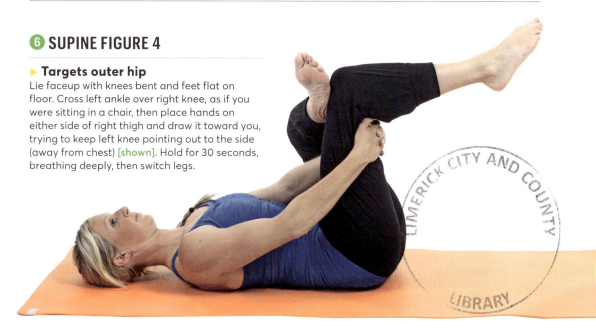

LIMERICK CITY AND COUNTY LIBRARY

CREDITS

COVER Dean Drobot/Shutterstock **2–3** SolisImages/Getty Images **4–5** Dougal Waters/Getty Images; PeopleImages/Getty Images; bowoedane/Shutterstock; Danny Bird/Kelsey Media **6–7** gettyimages/LiZhongfei **8–9** shutterstock/Dusan Petkovic **10–11** Maria Fuchs/Getty Images **12–13** Goran Bogicevic/Shutterstock **14–15** Vladeep/Shutterstock **16–17** Bojan Milinkov/Shutterstock; darwininin/Getty Images **18–19** Westend61/Getty Images **20–21** Michael Svoboda/Getty Images **22–23** vgajic/Getty Images; JGI/Jamie Grill/Getty Images **24–25** Tetra Images/Getty Images; Mike Harrington/Getty Images; Unitone Vector/Getty Images **26–27** fizkes/Getty Images **28–29** PeopleImages/Getty Images; Hiraman/Getty Images **30–31** HAO ZHANG/Getty Images **32–33** Matthew Ennis/Shutterstock **34–35** fizkes/Shutterstock **36–37** Zoe Hernandez (www.zoeella.com); grandriver/Getty Images; fizkes/Shutterstock **38–39** Dean Drobot/Shutterstock **40–41** johnkellerman/Getty Images; Maridav/Shutterstock **42–43** George Dolgikh/Shutterstock **44–45** Supreeya Chantalao/EyeEm/Getty Images **46–47** Courtesy of Superbands; Courtesy of FitBit **48–49** Courtesy of Bowflex; Tetiana Rostopira/Shutterstock; Microgen/Shutterstock; Courtesy of TrafficMaster; Courtesy of TRX **50–51** Bill Diodato/Getty Images **52–53** Simon Taylor/Kelsey Media; Danny Bird/Kelsey Media **54–55** Simon Taylor/Kelsey Media; Danny Bird/Kelsey Media; PeopleImages/Getty Images **56–57** TomFullum/Getty Images (2) **58–59** Eddie MacDonald/Kelsey Media; Danny Bird/Kelsey Media **60–61** Eddie MacDonald/Kelsey Media; Danny Bird/Kelsey Media **62–63** Mikhail Azarov/Getty Images **64–65** Danny Bird/Kelsey Media **66–67** Danny Bird/Kelsey Media; Phongthorn Hiranlikhit/EyeEm/Getty Images **68–69** inarik/Getty Images **70–71** Will Ireland/Kelsey Media; Hugh Threlfall/Kelsey Media; Danny Bird/Kelsey Media **72–73** CareyHope/Getty Images **74–75** Danny Bird/Kelsey Media; LightField Studios/Shutterstock **76–77** Mike Kemp/Getty Images **78–79** Will Ireland/Kelsey Media; Hugh Threlfall/Kelsey Media; Danny Bird/Kelsey Media; magenavi/Getty Images **80–81** Neustockimages/Getty Images; Eddie MacDonald/Kelsey Media; Danny Bird/Kelsey Media **82–83** Nastco/Getty Images; Eddie MacDonald/Kelsey Media; Danny Bird/Kelsey Media **84–85** nazarovsergey/Shutterstock **86–87** Henry Carter/Kelsey Media; herreid/Getty Images **88–89** pixdeluxe/Getty Images **90–91** Henry Carter/Kelsey Media; bowoedane/Shutterstock **92–93** Corey Jenkins/Getty Images **94–95** Klaus Vedfelt/Getty Images **96–97** Dougal Waters/Getty Images **98–99** vitapix/Getty Images **100–101** MoMo Productions/Getty Images **102–103** Maskot/Getty Images **104–105** CasarsaGuru/Getty Images **106–107** Luca Sage/Getty Images; Matt Lincoln/Getty Images **108–109** nortonrsx/Getty Images; Martin Novak/Getty Images **110–111** gradyreese/Getty Images **112–113** Cavan Images/Getty Images; andresr/Getty Images **114–115** The Image Bank/Getty Images; iStockphoto/Getty Images **116–117** Westend61/Getty Images **118–119** Henry Carter/Kelsey Media **120–121** djile/Shutterstock **122–123** Portra Images/Getty Images **124–125** Danny Bird/Kelsey Media **126–127** Danny Bird/Kelsey Media **128–129** Klaus Vedfelt/Getty Images **130–131** Danny Bird/Kelsey Media **132–133** FANDSrabutan/Getty Images; Kris Ubach and Quim Roser/Getty Images **134–135** gradyreese/Getty Images **136–137** Henry Carter/Kelsey Media **SPINE** bowoedane/Shutterstock **BACK COVER** Mike Harrington/Getty Images

SPECIAL THANKS TO CONTRIBUTING WRITERS

Nicole Dorsey, Brittany Risher, Deborah Skolnik

Before starting or modifying any fitness routine, consult with a licensed health professional who knows your personal medical history. Information in *20 Minutes, 4 Weeks, 1 Dynamite Body* is provided for awareness, education and general information. Health benefits of various fitness regimens and weight-loss strategies are the opinion of the author, and there may be differing views on many of the topics covered, including benefits, risk of injury and efficacy. This book is meant to inform the general reader and is not a substitute for advice from a fitness coach, licensed trainer and/or physician. The publishers assume no responsibility for risk of injury or death. Please consult a doctor if you feel any side effects from a fitness regimen.

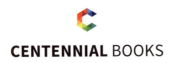

CENTENNIAL BOOKS

An Imprint of
Centennial Media, LLC
40 Worth St., 10th Floor
New York, NY 10013, U.S.A.

CENTENNIAL BOOKS is a trademark of Centennial Media, LLC

All rights reserved. No part of this publication may be reproduced,
stored in a retrieval system, or transmitted in any form or by any means
(including electronic, mechanical, photocopying, recording, or otherwise)
without prior written permission from the publisher.

ISBN 978-1-951274-65-8

Distributed by
Simon & Schuster, Inc.
1230 Avenue of the Americas
New York, NY 10020, U.S.A.

For information about custom editions, special sales
and premium and corporate purchases,
please contact Centennial Media at contact@centennialmedia.com.

Manufactured in China

© 2021 by Centennial Media, LLC

10 9 8 7 6 5 4 3 2 1

Publishers & Co-Founders Ben Harris, Sebastian Raatz
Editorial Director Annabel Vered
Creative Director Jessica Power
Executive Editor Janet Giovanelli
Features Editor Alyssa Shaffer
Deputy Editors Ron Kelly, Anne Marie O'Connor
Design Director Martin Elfers
Senior Art Director Pino Impastato
Art Directors Olga Jakim, Natali Suasnavas, Joseph Ulatowski
Copy/Production Patty Carroll, Angela Taormina
Assistant Art Director Jaclyn Loney
Photo Editor Jenny Veiga
Production Manager Paul Rodina
Production Assistant Alyssa Swiderski
Editorial Assistant Tiana Schippa
Sales & Marketing Jeremy Nurnberg